DR. ABBY GROSS

DR. ABBY GROSS

The Surgical Atlas of
Otology and Neuro-otology

Comprehensive Surgical Atlases in Otolaryngology and Head and Neck Surgery

Editor-in-Chief

K. J. Lee, M.D., F.A.C.S.

Director, Ear Research and Educational Center
Chairman, Education and Research Committee
Coordinator, Laser Surgery Center
President, Hospital of St. Raphael Medical Staff
Chairman, Medical Board
Hospital of St. Raphael
New Haven, Connecticut
Attending, Hospital of St. Raphael, Yale–New Haven Hospital, and Milford Hospital
New Haven and Milford, Connecticut
Consultant, Backus Hospital and Windham Community Hospital
Norwich and Willimantic, Connecticut
Assistant Clinical Professor, Department of Surgery
Yale University School of Medicine
New Haven, Connecticut

The Surgical Atlas of Otology and Neuro-otology
Eiji Yanagisawa, M.D., F.A.C.S., and Gale Gardner, M.D., F.A.C.S.

The Atlas of Head and Neck Surgery
Bruce W. Jafek, M.D., F.A.C.S., and Clarence T. Sasaki, M.D., F.A.C.S.

The Atlas of Aesthetic Facial Surgery
Douglas D. Dedo, M.D., F.A.C.S.

The Surgical Atlas of Airway and Facial Trauma
Robert H. Miller, M.D., F.A.C.S.

The Atlas of Cleft Lip and Cleft Palate Surgery
Howard W. Smith, M.D., D.M.D., F.A.C.S.

Foreword

In the five volumes in this series, the editors, contributors, and I have attempted to illustrate succinctly the current acceptable techniques in otolaryngology and head and neck surgery. When possible and appropriate, we have included alternative techniques for comparison.

I am greatly indebted to the editorial staff of Grune & Stratton, Inc., for their support and patience. I also thank the volume editors, contributors, and illustrators for enduring my numerous phone calls and letters. As usual, my wife and family have been most supportive.

In recognition of our teachers, the volume editors have dedicated these texts to their mentors.

K. J. Lee, M.D., F.A.C.S.
Editor-in-Chief

The Surgical Atlas of
Otology and Neuro-otology

Eiji Yanagisawa, M.D., F.A.C.S.

*Clinical Professor, Section of Otolaryngology
Department of Surgery
Yale University School of Medicine
Associate Chief, Section of Otolaryngology,
Department of Surgery
Hospital of St. Raphael
New Haven, Connecticut
Attending, Hospital of St. Raphael, Yale–New Haven
Hospital, and Milford Hospital
New Haven and Milford, Connecticut
Consultant, Meriden–Wallingford Hospital and
Waterbury Hospital
Meriden and Waterbury, Connecticut*

Gale Gardner, M.D., F.A.C.S.

*Clinical Associate Professor, Department of
Otolaryngology and Maxillofacial Surgery
University of Tennessee Center for Health Sciences
Memphis, Tennessee
Chairman, Department of Otolaryngology
Baptist Memorial Hospital
Memphis, Tennessee*

Illustrated by

David M. Bolinsky
New Haven, Connecticut

David Weyermann
Memphis, Tennessee

GRUNE & STRATTON
A Subsidiary of Harcourt Brace Jovanovich, Publishers
New York   London   Paris   San Diego   San Francisco   São Paulo   Sydney   Tokyo   Toronto

Library of Congress Cataloging in Publication Data
Main entry under title:

The surgical atlas of otology and neuro-otology.

(Comprehensive surgical atlases in otolaryngology and
head and neck surgery)
Includes bibliographies and index.
1. Ear—Surgery.   2. Auditory pathways—Surgery.
3. Labyrinth (Ear)—Surgery.   I. Yanagisawa, Eiji.
II. Gardner, Gale.   III. Series.   [DNLM: 1. Ear—Surgery—
Atlases.   WV 17 S961]
RF126.S97   1983   617.8′059   83-18565
ISBN 0-8089-1605-X

Grune & Stratton, Inc.
111 Fifth Avenue
New York, New York 10003

Distributed in the United Kingdom by
Grune & Stratton, Inc. (London) Ltd.
24/28 Oval Road, London NW 1

Library of Congress Catalog Number 83-18565
International Standard Book Number 0-8089-1605-X
Printed in the United States of America

——————— *To* ———————

John J. Shea, M.D.

Shea Clinic
Memphis, Tennessee

Who revived and refined stapedectomy in 1956,
thereby launching the modern era of micro-otologic surgery,
particularly surgery of the inner ear.

William F. House, M.D.

Clinical Professor, Department of Otolaryngology
University of Southern California School of Medicine
Research Director, House Ear Institute
Los Angeles, California

Who, beginning in 1959, applied microsurgery to the entire temporal bone,
developing the translabyrinthine and middle fossa
approaches for removal of acoustic tumors and
the surgical treatment of vertigo and facial nerve disorders.

Gale Gardner

Contents

This book intends to show residents and practicing otolaryngologists the basic surgical techniques used in commonly performed otologic and neuro-otologic procedures. Part I, edited by Dr. Eiji Yanagisawa, covers otology, and Part II, by Dr. Gale Gardner, covers neuro-otology. As in the other volumes in this series, the authors describe in each chapter the generally accepted technique or the technique of choice and illustrate it step-by-step. They follow the description with a discussion of various alternative techniques, some generally accepted and some controversial.

Preface to Part I

I strongly believe in the importance of documenting otologic surgery for teaching and better patient care. Hence I have included a brief description of the various methods of photographic documentation in Chapter 1.

I have made it a habit to sketch practically all of the otologic procedures I perform. Most of the illustrations used in my chapters have been redrawn by my medical illustrator from the rough sketches I made in my charts immediately following surgery.

At the end of most chapters I have described problems that are encountered both during and following surgery and their solutions. Most of these are based on observations I have made during the past 25 years of teaching otologic surgery. Many previously unpublished cases from my own clinical experience are included, particularly in Chapter 6 on ossicular reconstruction and Chapter 14 on surgery for congenital anomalies of the ear.

I would like to express my sincere gratitude to Dr. K. J. Lee for inviting me to edit Part I of this volume. I would also like to thank the contributors for the excellent job they did. My special appreciation goes to David M. Bolinsky, my medical illustrator and a member of the Department of Medical Illustration and Photography at Yale University School of Medicine, for his excellent, high-quality illustrations. He spent countless midnights and weekends with me, going over the illustrations and drawing them many times until we both were satisfied. Without his skill, dedication, patience, and understanding of ear surgery, this volume would never have materialized.

Special thanks also go to Dr. Myles L. Pensak, who not only coauthored several chapters but also spent many hours assisting me in preparing and correcting the manuscript, and to Drs. Kveton and Lee for their valuable contributions to this text.

Finally, I would like to acknowledge the support and encouragement of my family, office staff, and typists, particularly Karen Durr, without whom this volume would still remain unfinished.

Eiji Yanagisawa, M.D., F.A.C.S.

Preface to Part II

Although the emphasis of this text is on surgical technique, I have made an effort to stress its conceptual and fundamental elements, rather than those details that can be learned only in the dissection laboratory and in the operating room. For the sake of simplicity, all illustrations in this section are of the right temporal bone.

Although this material should be quite useful to the surgeon who is entering neuro-otologic surgery, no surgical atlas can substitute for actual surgical experience gained through a disciplined training program. Implicit in the presentation of a surgical atlas is the expectation that the reader must obtain basic surgical information from sources such as this and then proceed to acquire more advanced information from others and through personal surgical experience.

I would like to extend special thanks to David Weyermann, who illustrated the section on neuro-otology. He did so with great dedication and persistence, as well as artistic skill.

Gale Gardner, M.D., F.A.C.S.

Contributors

John F. Kveton, M.D. *Assistant Professor*
Department of Otolaryngology
St. Louis University School of Medicine
St. Louis, Missouri

Myles L. Pensak, M.D. *Fellow in Otology and Neuro-otology*
The Otology Group, P.C.
Nashville, Tennessee

I

Otology

Edited by
Eiji Yanagisawa

I

——Documentation of Otologic Surgery——

Otologic surgery can be documented by still, motion, and video photography. Photographic documentation is of great value for teaching, permanent records, and preoperative and postoperative evaluation of various otologic conditions.

STILL PHOTOGRAPHY

Still photography of ear surgery can be accomplished by utilizing the optical system of the Zeiss operating microscope. Since the microscope and the camera equipment can be easily covered with a sterile transparent plastic drape, microscopic photography is a preferred method of photography during microscopic ear surgery. Microscopic photography can be done with or without the use of a photoadapter.

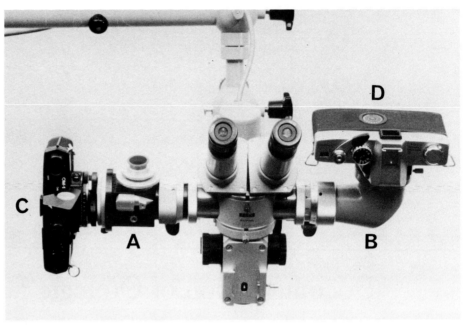

Figure 1-1

PHOTOGRAPHY WITH
A PHOTOADAPTER

Once the single-lens reflex (SLR) camera is interfaced to the Zeiss operating microscope by means of a photoadapter and a beam splitter, the system is immediately available for photography at any time during otologic surgery (Figure 1-1).

Figure 1-1 shows two different photoadapters attached to the beam splitter of the Zeiss operating microscope: (A) Telestill photoadapter by Design for Vision, (B) Zeiss photoadapter, (C) Olympus OM2 SLR camera with autowinder, and (D) Minolta SLR camera.

The following equipment is required: (1) Zeiss operating microscope, (2) Zeiss beam splitter (50:50 is preferred to 70:30 because the latter gives a poorer light for the surgeon), (3) photoadapter (Design for Vision, Zeiss, or Zeiss-Urban dual adapter), (4) adapter ring for SLR camera, and (5) automatic 35-mm SLR camera such as the Olympus OM2 or the Contax RTS.

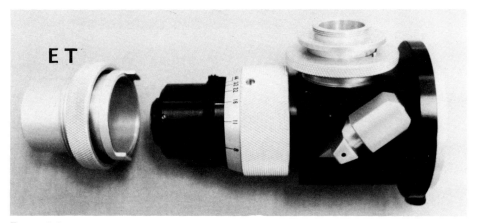

Figure 1-2

The Telestill photoadapter and its extension tube (ET) are shown in Figure 1-2. With the handle of the photoadapter in its 45° position, a focal *f* length of 137 mm assures proper TV focusing. When the handle is in the horizontal position, it provides a full-frame image for 35-mm cameras. The ET increases the distance between the TV camera and the beam splitter of the microscope, giving the surgeon more head room.

When the Olympus OM2 with autowinder and remote-control cable (1.2 or 5 m) or Contax RTS automatic camera with remote-control "across-the-room" shutter release is used, the camera itself need not be touched at all during photography. Vibrations of the camera are thus eliminated (Figures 1-1 and 1-3).

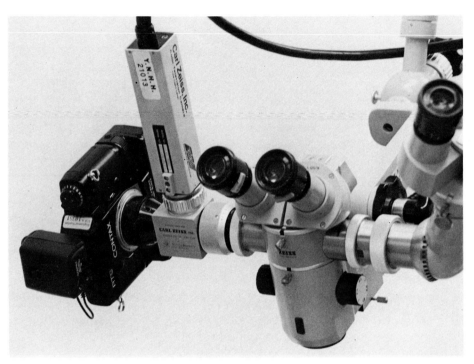

Figure 1-3

A Contax RTS SLR camera with this type of shutter release is shown in Figure 1-3 attached to the Zeiss-Urban dual photoadapter. Note that a miniature video camera (Carl Zeiss) is also attached to the same photoadapter. Simultaneous still and video photography is possible with this system.

High Speed Ektachrome Tungsten film ASA 160 is used. The ASA dial on the camera is set at 320, and the film is push-processed at ASA 320. If an electronic flash is utilized, High Speed Ektachrome Daylight ASA 200 film is used.

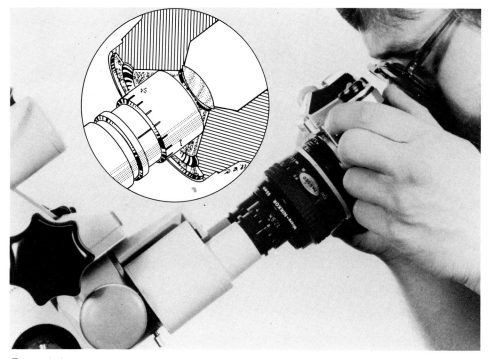

Figure 1-4

PHOTOGRAPHY WITHOUT A PHOTOADAPTER

This is known as the *macrolens technique,* in which the macrolens of the camera is placed over an eyepiece of the microscope (Figure 1-4). The image should be in focus through the viewfinder of the camera. The insert in Figure 1-4 shows that the recessed front housing of the macrolens prevents direct contact of the lens surface with the eyepiece of the microscope.

The middle-ear and mastoid structures can be simply photographed through the eyepiece of the operating microscope by using the SLR camera with a macrolens technique.

The following equipment is required: (1) Zeiss operating microscope, (2) "aperture-preferred" automatic 35-mm SLR camera such as Nikon FE, Pentax ME, Olympus OM2, OM10, Minolta X-700 or XG, and (3) 50-mm macrolens. Ektachrome Tungsten film ASA 160 is used and pushed to 320.

In this technique the camera is set at infinity with the lens maximally open (usually $f3.5$). The eyepiece of the microscope is set at 0. The structure to be photographed is focused through the microscope first. The microscope knob is tightened. The macrolens of the camera is placed on the eyepiece of the microscope. The structure is then focused *through the viewfinder of the camera* and the pictures taken (Figure 1-4).

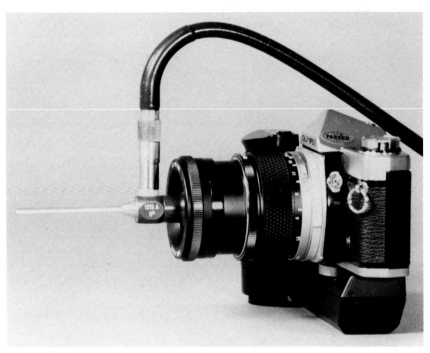

Figure 1-5

TELESCOPIC PHOTOGRAPHY

The Hopkins 4.0-mm otoscopic telescope can be used for still photography of ear surgery. The telescope is gas-sterilized or soaked in sterilizing solution. The following equipment is required: (1) Hopkins telescope 1215A (4.0 mm) shown attached to the 100-mm lens of the Olympus OM2 camera with an autowinder in Figure 1-5 or 1218A (2.7 mm), (2) dual-mode flash and examining light system (Karl Storz No. 558 or 559 CA), (3) quick connect camera adapter, (4) Olympus OM2 SLR camera with an autowinder and a 1–9 (or 1–12) focusing screen, (5) 100-mm Zuiko lens, and (6) Ektachrome Daylight film ASA 200 (Figure 1-5).

The tip of the telescope is dipped in sterile warm water and wiped to prevent fogging during photography. A series of pictures are taken at different depths by depressing the shutter release of the autowinder. The autowinder eliminates the necessity of removing the camera from the operating field for each advancement of the film.

MOTION PICTURES

The motion pictures taken with a 16-mm movie camera give a sharp, clear image of the structures of the middle ear and mastoid. Movie documentation is ideal for showing in a large auditorium.

Motion pictures can be taken by attaching a 16-mm movie camera such as the House-Urban camera (Figure 1-6) or the Beaulieu R-16 camera (shown attached to a Zeiss cineadapter, F137, in Figure 1-7) to the Zeiss operating microscope by a photoadapter and a beam splitter (Figure 1-5). Certain Super 8 movie cameras with a C-mount coupler can also be used.

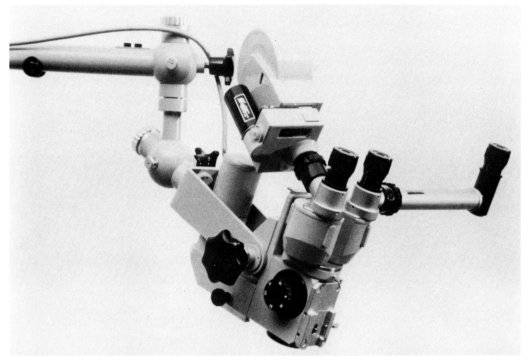

Figure 1-6

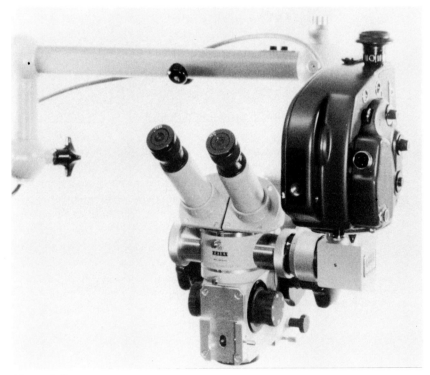

Figure 1-7

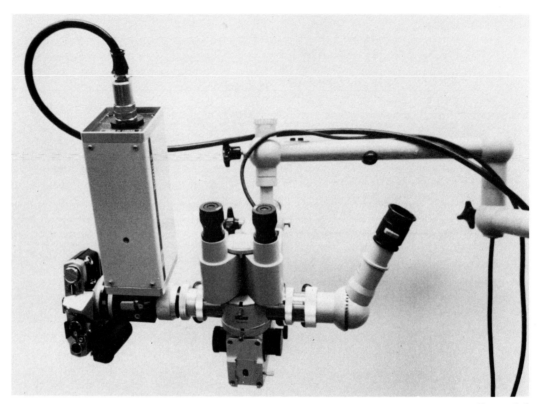

Figure 1-8

VIDEOTAPE RECORDING

Thanks to recent technologic advances and miniaturization of the television camera, it has become possible to televise and videotape otologic surgery relatively simply and inexpensively (except for the inital cost of setting up the equipment). The following equipment is required: (1) Zeiss operating microscope, (2) Zeiss beam splitter, (3) photoadapter (Design for Vision, Zeiss, or Zeiss-Urban), (4) video camera [Hitachi color HV9017 (shown attached to a Telestill photoadapter in Figure 1-8), Zeiss-Urban, Circon], and (5) remote foot control for videotape recording (Figures 1-3 and 1-8).

DISCUSSION

One of the major advantages of microscopic photography (see description of Figures 1-1–1-3) with the use of a photoadapter is the ease of photography. While performing the operation, the surgeon can photograph the ear at any time with minimal interference to the procedure. Other advantages are that the ear can be photographed at different magnifications (6×–40×), cropping and enlargement of the finished slide for lectures are not necessary when taken at higher magnifications, and video and movie photography can conveniently and simultaneously be done with relative ease through the dual adapter (Zeiss-Urban).

Some of the disadvantages are that the photoadapter and a beam splitter are expensive, the depth of field is very shallow, particularly at high magnification, and meticulous refocusing is necessary with each magnification. Moreover, it is almost impossible to obtain perfect focus of all portions of the ear canal, mastoid, and middle ear in the same picture.

Photographs taken by the non-photoadapter-assisted technique (Figure 1-4) are of surprisingly good quality, but the results are not always predictable. The macrolens technique is the least expensive method of microscopic photography. Some of the disadvantages are that it is difficult to hold the camera still on the eyepiece of the microscope, the procedure is interrupted because the picture must be taken either by an assistant or even by the surgeon, the success rate is not as high as the technique with the photoadapter, and a bright illumination and a high-speed color film are required.

Telescopic photography offers several advantages over microscopic photography. Microscopic photography offers only a portion of the tympanic membrane for transcanal procedures because of the tortuosity of the ear canal and the prominence of the anterior bony canal wall. Since the tip of the telescope can be advanced beyond the narrow isthmus of the ear canal, it can demonstrate the entire tympanic membrane or wide areas of the middle-ear space. The wide-angle view of the Hopkins optic provides an almost infinite depth of field so that the entire tympanic membrane can be seen in focus.

Some of the disadvantages include the facts that the equipment is expensive, the lens constantly fogs during photography, and there is some distortion of the image of the tympanic membrane and other small structures of the middle ear as a result of the wide-angle effect of the telescopic lens. In addition, it is difficult to sterilize the instrument for use in the operating room, and the procedure is interrupted because the picture must be taken by either the surgeon or an assistant.

In the procedures described in reference to Figures 1-6 and 1-7, some of the disadvantages are that motion pictures are generally inconvenient and technically difficult because of the bulky size of the camera and their use is time-consuming. Also, film is expensive, and splicing and editing are costly. Although it is easy to transfer movie pictures to videotapes, it is extremely difficult and costly to transfer TV images to movie film.

One advantage of videotaping (Figure 1-8) is that it permits live viewing by interns, residents, nurses, and other operating room personnel. In addition, there is no interference with surgery; instant replay is possible; electronic editing can be done without splicing; duplication is easy; and videotapes are reasonably priced and reusable and can immediately be used for teaching, conferences, and permanent records.

The disadvantages of videotaping are that initial equipment is expensive, the procedure is time-consuming, and electronic editing is costly and time-consuming. Moreover, showing videotapes in a large auditorium requires costly multiple TV monitors or a giant TV screen, equipment rapidly becomes obsolete, high-intensity illumination is required for a TV camera, there is incompatibility between different makes of equipment, and technical expertise is often required in the operating room.

In spite of these disadvantages, the author feels that videotape recording is the most valuable method of documentation and teaching of otologic surgery.

REFERENCES

1. Buckingham, R. A.: Photography of the ear. In: Otolaryngology, Vol. 1, G. M. English (Ed). Harper & Row, New York, chap. 58, 1981.

2. Chole, R. A.: Photography of the Tympanic Membrane, a New Method. *Arch. Otolaryngol.*, 106:230–231, 1980.

3. Hawke, M.: Telescopic Otoscopy and Photography of the Tympanic Membrane. *J. Otolaryngol.*, 11:35–39, 1982.

4. Hughes, G. B., Yanagisawa, E., Dickins, J. R. E., *et al.*: Microscopic Otologic Photography Using a Standard 35mm Camera. *Am. J. Otol.*, 2:243–247, 1981.

5. Lundborg, T. and Linzander, S.: The Otomicroscopic Observation and Its Clinical Application. *Acta Otolaryngol.* (Stockh.) (suppl.) 266:3–36, 1970.

6. Yanagisawa, E.: Effective Photography in Otolaryngology—Head and Neck Surgery: Tympanic Membrane Photography. *Otolaryngol. Head Neck Surg.* 90:399–407, 1982.

2
──────Myringotomy──────

K. J. Lee
John F. Kveton

TECHNIQUES

Myringotomy and pressure-equalizing (PE) tube insertion is most easily performed under general anesthesia in infants and children, whereas local anesthesia is effective for most adults (Figure 2-1). If local anesthesia is used, 1 ml of 1% lidocaine (Xylocaine) with epinephrine 1:100,000 is injected into the canal wall skin at four to six equal positions at the chondro-osseous junction. This is best accomplished with an angled No. 25–30 gauge, 1½-inch needle to provide optimal visibility while injecting. The bevel of the needle should abutt the canal wall bone (under the periosteum). To reduce pain, infiltration should begin in previously anesthetized regions after the first injection. Injection should be

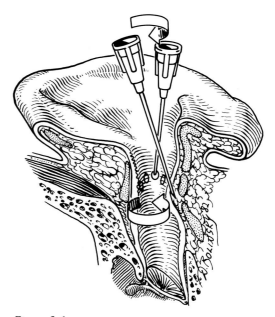

Figure 2-1

13

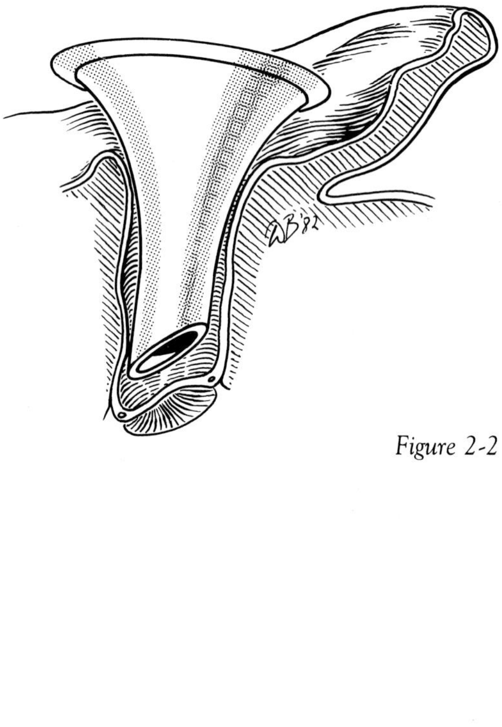

done slowly so that the solution does not enter the middle ear. Anesthetic in the middle ear can produce vertigo or delayed facial paralysis. Improper patient positioning can lead to inadequate visualization of the tympanic membrane. Placement of a shoulder roll allows easier rotation of the head, thus maximizing exposure of the anterior tympanum.

With the use of No. 5 or 7 Baron's suction, a wax loop, and an alligator forceps for adherent fragments, the external canal is cleared of all debris and cerumen. Abrasion of the thin anterior canal wall skin should be avoided, since bleeding will obstruct the view of the tympanic membrane. Minute debris is then irrigated from the canal with normal saline or iodine solution.

An oval, beveled speculum of largest possible diameter is inserted into the external canal with the bevel anteriorly (Figure 2-2). This snug speculum fit will provide optimal visualization as well as reduce canal wall trauma. The anterior canal wall bulge, a frequent trouble spot, can be easily negotiated by tilting the speculum posteriorly when the bulge is encountered, advancing toward the tympanic membrane, and then tilting anteriorly.

Figure 2-2

The tympanic membrane is inspected and landmarks identified. Visualization of the umbo provides orientation, particularly when a thickened or bulging membrane obscures normal landmarks. This is especially important in young children under mask anesthesia when fear of airway obstruction prompts the surgeon to move quickly. The tympanic membrane should be examined for perforation, retraction, myringosclerosis, or monomembrane formation to ensure PE tube placement (Figure 2-3) in a healthy portion of the drum.

The type of PE tube used and its position on the tympanic membrane determines the duration of middle-ear ventilation. Epithelial migration of the squamous portion of the drum, thought to be responsible for tube extrusion, radiates from the umbo. This migration is fastest in the posteroinferior and anteroinferior quadrants, followed by the posterosuperior and anterosuperior quadrants, respectively. The anterosuperior quadrant is thus the optimal location for prolonged tube position. Tube insertion in the posterosuperior quadrant obviously is contraindicated because of location of the ossicles. The inferior quadrants may be used for shorter periods of middle-ear ventilation and are the most accessible. Bobbin-type, uniformly flanged PE tubes (Figure 2-3A) migrate off the tympanic membrane slower than the angled (B) or arrow (C) inner-flanged tubes.

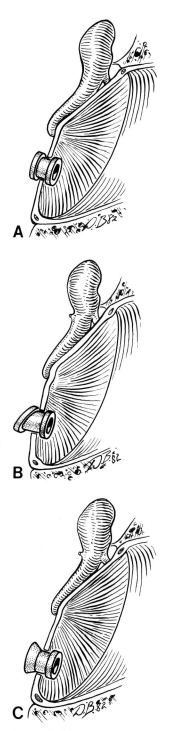

Figure 2-3

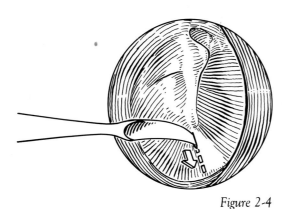

Figure 2-4

A straight or angled myringotomy knife is inserted into the tympanic membrane and the myringotomy incision is lengthened by a slight sawing motion of the knife (Figure 2-4). The direction of the myringotomy incision is important. A radially oriented incision parallels the direction of epithelial migration, whereas the circumferential incision is perpendicular to it. Epithelial accumulation is thus greater with a circumferential incision, producing a faster extrusion rate.[2] Bleeding from the tympanic membrane is usually minimal, but if troublesome, it may be controlled with cotton pledgelets saturated with epinephrine solution (1:1000). Profuse bleeding at myringotomy may be due to an aberrantly located jugular bulb. Packing the middle ear with Gelfoam and the external canal with Nugauze will tamponade the hemorrhage.

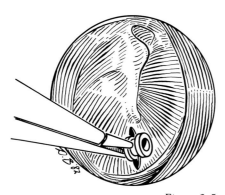

Figure 2-5

After myringotomy any fluid, mucus, or pus in the middle ear is suctioned with a No. 5 Baron's suction (Figure 2-5). If secretions are thick and tenacious, saline irrigation with a No. 7 Baron's suction is helpful. The outer flange of the PE tube, opposite the leading edge, is now grasped with an alligator forceps and introduced into the external canal without touching the canal wall. In a small canal the tube should be grasped by the inner flange. A PE tube insertor may also be used.

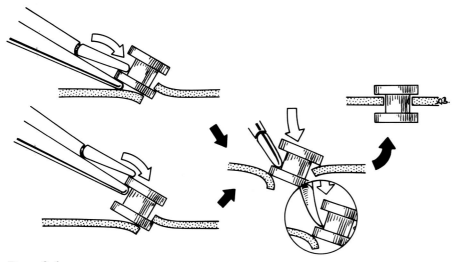

Figure 2-6

The leading edge of the inner flange is then en-
gaged in the myringotomy incision (Figure 2-6). It
is important to make sure that the anterior edge of
the inner flange is within the incision. With the
use of the myringotomy knife or the tip of the alligator forceps, firm pressure is applied to the junction of the shaft and the inner flange in an anter-
omedial direction to "pop" the posterior portion of
the inner flange under the posterior edge of the
myringotomy site, thus inserting the tube. This
method works best for firm polyethylene tubes. Soft
PE tubes such as silicone are more difficult to insert
and require a slightly larger myringotomy incision.
Occasionally a PE tube is lost in the middle ear on
insertion. Careful retrieval should be attempted
through the myringotomy, with attention to the
chance of ossicular disruption. If necessary, a tympanomeatal flap should be raised to retrieve a tube
lodged in the posterior tympanum.

After placement of the tube, patency is assured by clearing the tubal orifice of any blood or mucus by suctioning with the thumb off the suction vent. This prevents suctioning the tube out of the myringotomy incision. Sterile saline can be used to irrigate the orifice until clear. Epinephrine-saturated cotton pledgets will control persistent bleeding around the tube. If tubal patency remains in question as a result of continuous drainage from the middle ear, otic drops are administered in the immediate postoperative period. The author has found that the use of Neodecadron Ophthalmic drops in this situation avoids the burning sensation of which many patients complain when regular otic drops are used.

DISCUSSION

TYPES OF PE TUBES

In general, PE tubes are made of Teflon, polyethylene, silicone, or stainless steel. Extrusion rates vary with the material and are most rapid with silicone, followed by polyethylene and Teflon mesh, respectively.[4] Inner diameters of PE tubes range from 2.3 to 5.0 mm. There are over a dozen types of PE tubes marketed, and tube selection is most often a matter of personal preference.

Permanent PE tubes differ in design as well as method of insertion. The Per-Lee tube is prototypic, consisting of an angled, wide inner flange and a long shaft. Absence of an outer flange on permanent tubes inhibits extrusion that occurs by epithelial accumulation under the outer flange. The Silverstein permanent aeration tube has an inner flange at 90° from the shaft, whereas the Goode T-Tube replaces the inner flange with a "T-arm" for ease of insertion and extraction. Placement of the permanent tubes involves elevation of a tympanomeatal flap and insertion of the tube medial to the bony annulus or malleus. The Silverstein tube is inserted into a hole drilled into the facial recess under the tympanomeatal flap in the region of the round window anterior to the facial nerve. The Goode T-

Tube is inserted directly into a myringotomy incision by closing the T-arm with an alligator forceps and then releasing it after insertion through the myringotomy incision. Many surgeons now trim or notch the Per-Lee tube inner flange and insert it directly into a myringotomy incision.

EXTRACTION AND REINSERTION

Pressure-equalization tube extraction is indicated in cases of chronic drainage or prolonged intubation of the middle ear. Chronic discharge, whether serous, mucoid, or bloody, is the most common late complication of PE tube insertion. Granulation tissue formation in the middle ear or on the tympanic membrane is the usual cause, especially in the presence of recurrent, bloody discharge. Extraction usually can be accomplished by prying the inner flange out of the myringotomy site with a small hook on the outer flange and removing the tube with an alligator forceps. The tympanic membrane and myringotomy site should then be carefully inspected for granulation tissue or cholesteatoma. Middle-ear exploration is mandatory with removal of any cholesteatomatous debris. Permanent PE tubes must be removed by elevation of a tympanomeatal flap unless the tube was placed directly into the myringotomy site. The Goode T-Tube may be directly extracted since the T-arm folds on itself with lateral traction on the shaft.

Chronic perforations of the tympanic membrane occur in less than 2 percent of intubated ears, whereas retraction or monomembrane formation occurs more often.[3]

Persistent middle-ear effusion after extraction or expulsion of a PE tube is an indication for reinsertion. Reimplantation preferably should occur at another site on the drum, since use of the same site increases the risk of permanent perforation, retraction, or monomembrane formation. In some situations the PE tube must be reinserted into the same site after it has been debrided of any squamous epithelium to prevent introduction of squamous epithelium into the middle ear.

REFERENCES

1. Alberti, P. N. R. M.: Epithelial Migration on the Tympanic Membrane. *J. Laryngol. Otol.*, 78:808–816, 1964.
2. Gibb, A. G. Long Term Assessment of Ventilation Tubes. *J. Laryngol. Otol.*, 94:39–51, 1980.
3. Hughes, L. A., Warder, F. R., and Hudson, W. R.: Complications of Tympanostomy Tubes. *Arch. Otolaryngol.*, 100:151–154, 1974.
4. Pappas, J. J.: Middle Ear Ventilation Tubes. *Laryngoscope*, 84:1098–1116, 1974.

3

Meatoplasty and Canalplasty

INTRACTABLE EXTERNAL OTITIS

Severe stenosing chronic external otitis that has resisted all usual forms of medical treatment should be surgically treated. The surgical procedure recommended by Paparella and Saunders is highly effective.

PAPARELLA-SAUNDERS[5,6] TECHNIQUE

The ear canal is completely stenosed by chronically inflamed, markedly thickened skin (Figure 3-1).

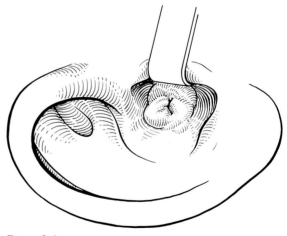

Figure 3-1

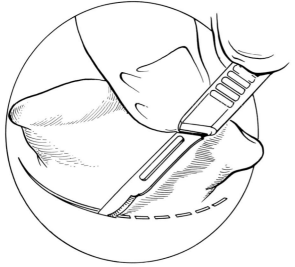

A postauricular incision is made (Figure 3-2).

Figure 3-2

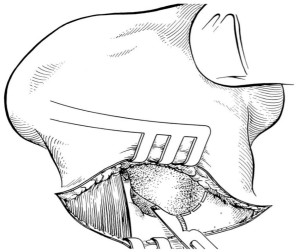

The posterior membranous canal is completely transected at the level of the cortex of the mastoid (Figure 3-3).

Figure 3-3

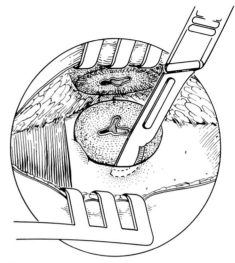

The diseased skin of the ear canal is excised by use of sharp knife blades (Figure 3-4), and canal skin is elevated.

Figure 3-4

All diseased skin is then removed from the ear canal (Figure 3-5). When there is marked bony exostosis, the diseased skin may have to be removed piecemeal. Care should be taken so as not to traumatize the tympanic membrane.

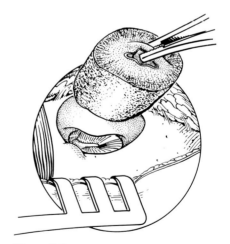

Figure 3-5

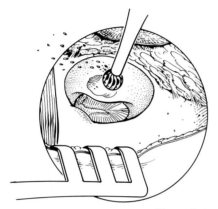

The bony ear canal is enlarged by using cutting burrs to its maximum so that the entire tympanic membrane can be seen (Figure 3-6). Care should be exercised to avoid entry into the mastoid air-cell system.

Figure 3-6

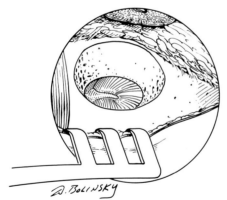

The squamous epithelium of the outer layer of the tympanic membrane is then removed (Figure 3-7).

Figure 3-7

A meatoplasty is performed by excision of a through-and-through elliptical wedge of conchal skin and cartilage (Figure 3-8).

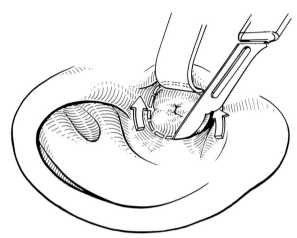

Figure 3-8

A plug of diseased skin including an ellipse of conchal cartilage is removed (Figure 3-9).

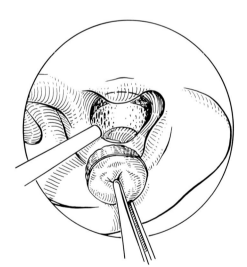

Figure 3-9

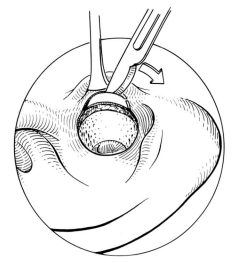

The remnants of the anterior cartilaginous canal skin are removed up to the tragus (Figure 3-10).

Figure 3-10

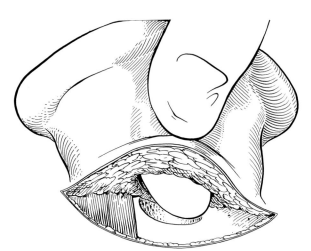

The meatus should be large enough to easily permit the entrance of an index finger (Figure 3-11).

Figure 3-11

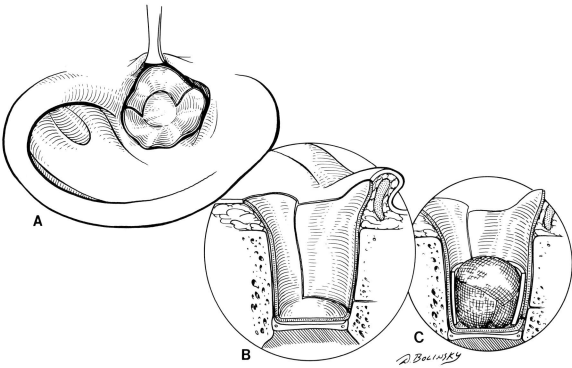

Figure 3-12

Split-thickness skin grafts are taken from the upper medial surface of the arm or from the lower abdomen. Two grafts are used: one for the tympanic membrane and the posterior canal wall, and the other for the anterior canal wall. The posterior graft is carefully placed against the tympanic membrane so that the distal end of the graft reflects onto the adjacent anterior canal wall of the anterior annulus (Figure 3-12A). The lateral part of the graft extends back against the posterior bony and cartilaginous canal, up to the conchal skin of the auricle (Figure 3-12B). The anterior skin graft covers the rest of the bony and cartilaginous canal. The ear canal is packed by use of a double-packing technique (Figure 3-12C).

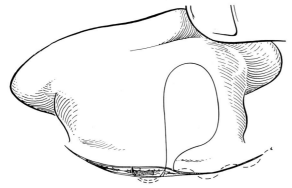

Figure 3-13

After the first medial pack is placed, the postauricular incision is closed (Figure 3-13).

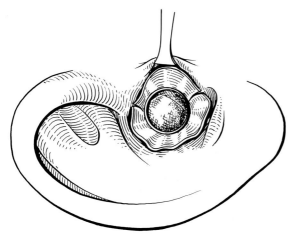

Figure 3-14

The lateral portions of the anterior and posterior skin grafts are carefully placed edge to edge up to the conchal incision posteriorly and up to the tragal incision anteriorly (Figure 3-14). Any excess skin is removed.

Fine catgut sutures are used to secure the grafts (Figure 3-15).

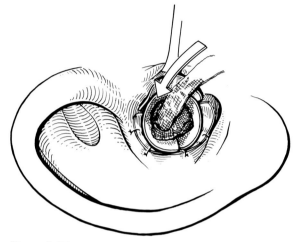

Figure 3-15

The outer pack is applied through the ear canal (Figure 3-16). The packings are kept for 2 weeks postoperatively.

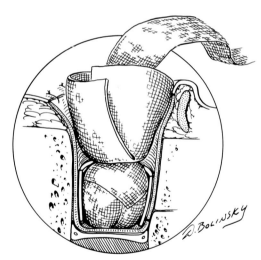

Figure 3-16

ALTERNATIVE PROCEDURES

The full-thickness skin graft technique, described below, is a modification of the technique described by Paparella and Saunders. The procedure is essentially the same, except that the postauricular full-thickness skin is used instead of the split-thickness skin. The full-thickness skin helps to partially fill the defect caused by the wedge resection of the concha. Removal of the postauricular elliptical skin retracts the auricle backward, increasing the patency of the canal. The use of this skin also eliminates the need for obtaining the skin from a different anatomic site.

Another departure from the Paparella-Saunders technique is that the squamous layer of the edematous tympanic membranes is not removed. The edematous, thickened membrane returns to normal after the surgery. The maintenance of an epithelial layer will help to prevent blunting of the anterior and inferior tympanic sulcus. Also in cases where the anterior canal skin is not heavily involved with inflammatory changes, the anterior canal skin is left in place.

Full-Thickness Skin Graft Technique

An elliptical skin incision is made (Figure 3-17). A small stab wound is made across the midportion of the incisions to facilitate an anatomically correct closure.

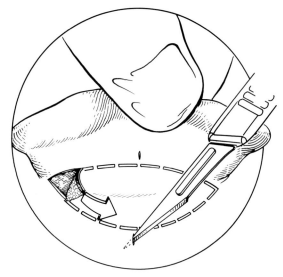

Figure 3-17

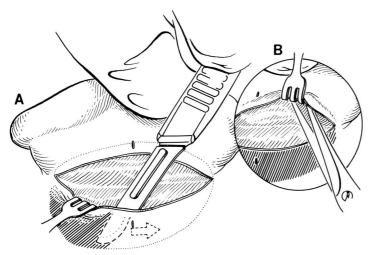

Figure 3-18

The posterior skin flap is generously undermined (Figure 3-18A). The anterior skin flap is undermined (Figure 3-18B). Note that only minimal undermining is done to ensure skin closure without dead space.

Upon completion of the canalplasty and meatoplasty, the incision is closed (Figure 3-19).

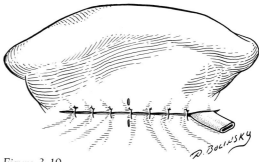

Figure 3-19

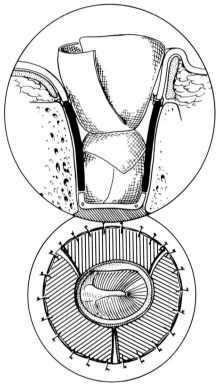

When all the canal skin is involved with the disease process, it is removed and replaced with full-thickness skin grafts (Figure 3-20).

Figure 3-20

When the anterior wall skin is minimally involved with the disease process, it is left intact (Figure 3-21). All exposed bone is covered with full-thickness skin grafts.

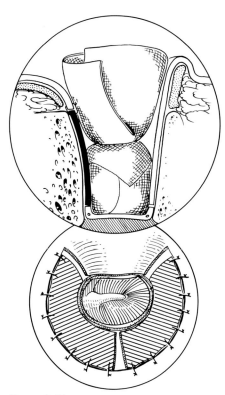

Figure 3-21

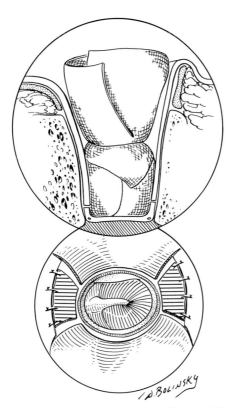

Figure 3-22

Körner's Flap Technique

In this technique, the posterior canal skin is thinned, a large piece of conchal cartilage is excised, and the flap is laid over the posterior bony canal. The anterior canal skin is also preserved and laid over the bony canal after the bony canal is maximally enlarged by drilling. Full-thickness skin grafts are placed superiorly and inferiorly to cover the exposed bone and subcutaneous tissues.

Both anterior and posterior canal skin flaps are repositioned after maximal widening of the bony canal (Figure 3-22). Full-thickness skin grafts are in place.

EXOSTOSIS OF THE EAR CANAL

TRANSMEATAL APPROACH

This approach is used for a small osteoma of the ear canal. An osteoma of the ear canal can be removed by a curet when it is attached to the ear canal with a relatively narrow base (Figure 3-23).

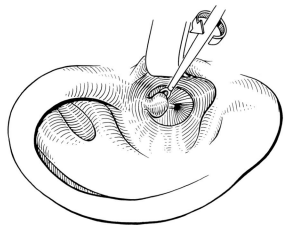

Figure 3-23

After removal of the osteoma, the rough bony surface may be smoothened by a curet or a drill (Figure 3-24A, B).

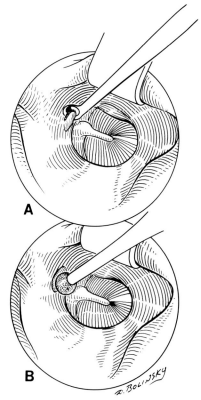

Figure 3-24

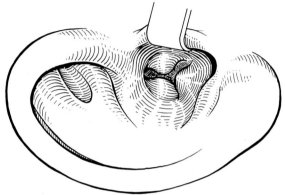
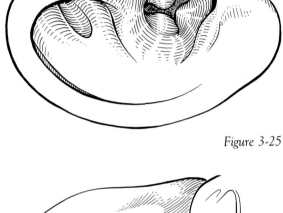

POSTAURICULAR APPROACH

This approach is used for extensive or multiple exostoses of the ear canal. Although the endaural approach can be used, it is technically more difficult, and the chances of preserving the skin flaps are smaller.

Endaural inspection shows large exostoses arising from the anterior, posterior, and superior canal walls (Figure 3-25).

Figure 3-25

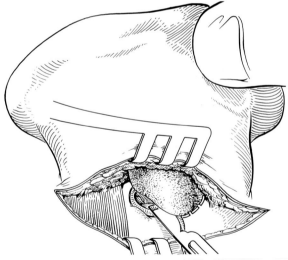

The posterior membranous canal wall is incised at the level of the cortex of the mastoid from the 12 o'clock to 6 o'clock positions, and the mastoid cortex and the ear canal are exposed (Figure 3-26).

Figure 3-26

The anterior part of the self-retaining retractor is repositioned to include the lateral aspect of the incised membranous canal wall. In this way, all exostoses including the anterior wall are well visualized (Figure 3-27).

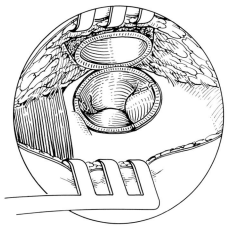

Figure 3-27

The skin over the posterior and inferior exostoses is reflected medially. Longitudinal incisions are made in the grooves between the exostoses (Figure 3-28).

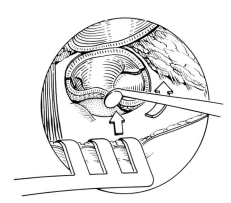

Figure 3-28

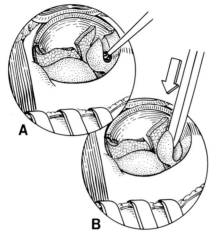

After the skin covering the inferior exostosis is elevated medially, a small groove is made at the base of the exostosis with a small cutting burr (Figure 3-29A).

With the use of a small chisel, the exostosis is then carefully removed (Figure 3-29B).

Figure 3-29

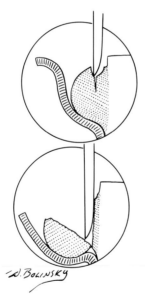

Removal of the exostosis is performed under microscopic observation (Figure 3-30). It is important to make a groove first in order to prevent injury to the facial nerve as the posterior canal wall may be cracked by chiseling. When done carefully, this is a very safe and effective technique for removing exostosis or osteoma of the ear canal.

Figure 3-30

The posterior canal skin is then elevated further (Figure 3-31).

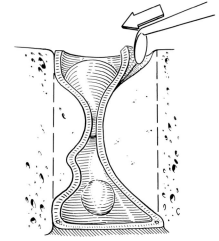

Figure 3-31

The exostosis is removed from lateral to medial position by a small-sized cutting burr (Figure 3-32).

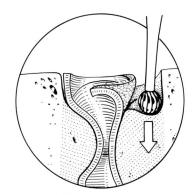

Figure 3-32

The posterior canal wall is thinned (Figure 3-33). However, the mastoid air cells must not be exposed, as this would be a cause of future fistula between the mastoid and the ear canal or formation of a cholesteatoma.

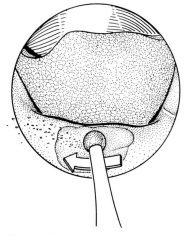

Figure 3-33

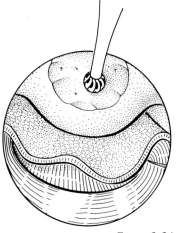

The anterior canal skin is elevated, and the exostosis is excised with a drill (Figure 3-34).

Figure 3-34

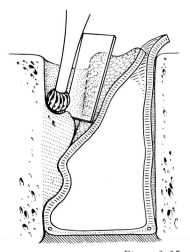

In order to protect the flap, a piece of thin Silastic sheet or Gelfilm is used (Figure 3-35). Only the diamond burr should be used in the medial portion of the ear canal to protect the flaps and the tympanic membrane.

Figure 3-35

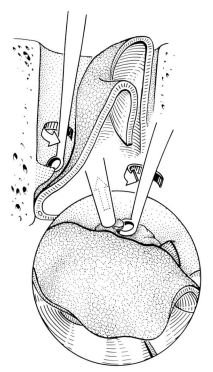

The most medial portion of the exostosis can often be safely and effectively removed with a small-sized Lempert curet (Figure 3-36). The skin is reflected back over the expanded canal wall. Bone should be removed until the anterior annular sulcus is visualized.

Figure 3-36

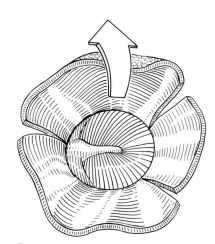

After the complete excision of the exostoses, the canal skin flaps are brought back to cover the enlarged bony canal (Figure 3-37).

Figure 3-37

The ear canal is then packed with a rosebud-type pack medially, and Vaseline (petrolatum) gauze is encased in a surgical rayon sleeve laterally (Figure 3-38).

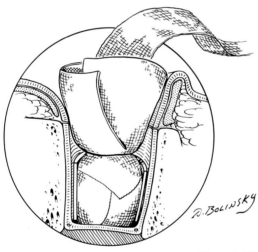

Figure 3-38

"MALIGNANT" EXTERNAL OTITIS

Also referred to as *necrotizing external otitis* (Chandler), this is a serious infection (*Pseudomonas aeruginosa*) with a high mortality rate that occurs in the elderly diabetic. The pathognomonic sign is the presence of active granulation tissue in the floor of the external auditory canal at the junction of its osseous and cartilaginous portions.

Treatment should consist of local debridement and systemic administration of carbenicillin and gentamicin. If the diagnosis is confirmed, surgical treatment must be carried out at once to prevent serious complications. If the diagnosis is made early, the procedure described here should be effective. If the diagnosis is delayed and *facial paralysis* is noted, a more extensive procedure may be necessary. Wide surgical debridement, including radical mastoidectomy, total parotidectomy, excision of the condyle and ascending ramus of the mandible, and—occasionally—sacrifice of the facial nerve may be necessary.[1,2]

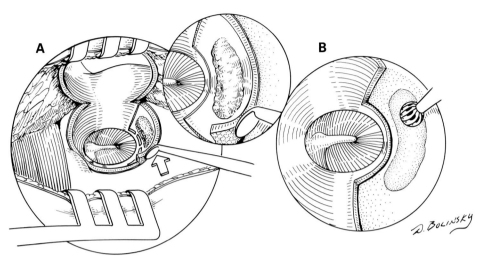

Figure 3-39

Through the postauricular approach, granulation tissue in the floor of the ear canal is exposed (Figure 3-39A). Two vertical incisions with a wide margin from the diseased tissues are made and connected medially just lateral to the tympanic membrane. The meatal skin is then removed with the diseased tissues. The bony ear canal is carefully examined with the operating microscope, and the involved bone is drilled away until healthy bone can be visualized (Figure 3-39B).

The skin defect of the ear canal is covered with a thin full-thickness skin graft taken from the postauricular area (Figure 3-40). The postauricular incision is closed, and the canal is packed with antibiotic soaked gauze.

MEATOPLASTY COMBINED WITH MASTOID SURGERY

See Chapter 13, on radical and modified radical mastoidectomy.

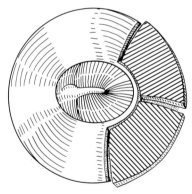

Figure 3-40

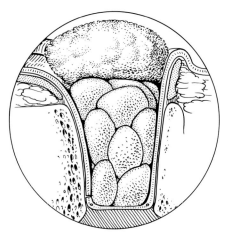

Figure 3-41

PACKING TECHNIQUES

The reconstructed ear canal and meatus should be carefully and meticulously packed. Undue pressure on the grafted skin or fascia should be avoided. To prevent postoperative infections, packing should be either soaked or impregnated with topical antibiotic ointment. The tympanic membrane should be first covered with pieces of Gelfoam before any type of packing is placed. Many different techniques are shown below.

The entire ear canal is packed with antibiotic soaked Gelfoam and a cotton ball (Sheehy) (Figure 3-41).

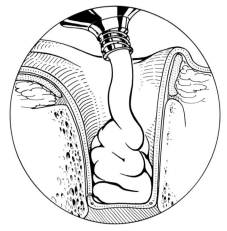

Figure 3-42

The canal is filled with antibiotic ointment (Glasscock) (Figure 3-42).

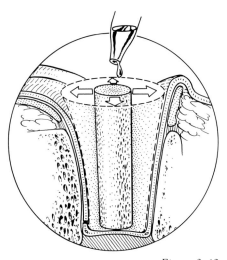

Figure 3-43

The canal is packed with Merocel fibersponge (Pope ear wick—Richards) (Figure 3-43); when moistened, this pack expands to fill the entire ear canal.

A surgical rayon sleeve (Owens nonadherent surgical dressing by American Cyanamid Company) is applied, into which elastic sponge packing or ½-inch petrolatum (Vaseline) gauze is placed (Figure 3-44).

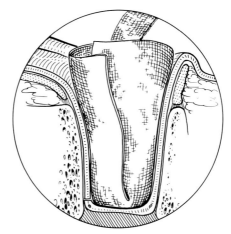

Figure 3-44

Telfa surgical dressing (Kendall) is rolled to fill the ear canal (K. J. Lee) (Figure 3-45).

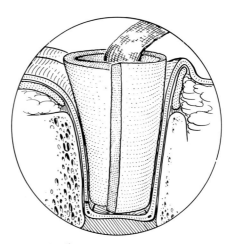

Figure 3-45

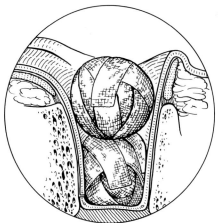

The double-packing technique by Paparella, consisting of the medial and lateral rosebud packings, is applied (Figure 3-46). The first pack, placed in the bony portion of the canal through the postauricular exposure, consists of strips of surgical rayon followed by cotton soaked in topical steroid. The second pack is applied endaurally. These packs are removed 2 weeks later.

Figure 3-46

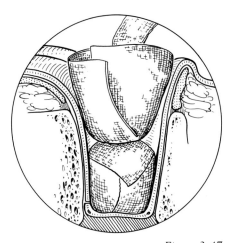

The double-packing technique by Yanagisawa is applied (Figure 3-47). The medial pack consists of three surgical rayon sheets in which approximately 4 cm of ½-inch petrolatum (Vaseline) gauze is packed. The outer packing consists of surgical rayon sleeve into which antibiotic impregnated ½-inch Vaseline gauze is placed to give "gentle" pressure against the meatal skin or flap. Prior to the placement of the medial pack, the skin graft is protected by a piece of ¼-inch rubber drain.

Figure 3-47

The ear canal is packed with ½-inch Vaseline gauze (Figure 3-48). This technique is not recommended because the granulation tissues grow into the gauze. When the packing is removed, the grafts may come with the packing, resulting in postoperative stenosis.

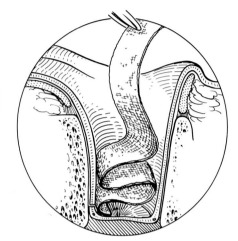

Figure 3-48

A thin silastic sheet covers the grafted skin of the canal before the packing is placed (Figure 3-49). This will prevent accidental removal of the skin grafts when the packing is removed.

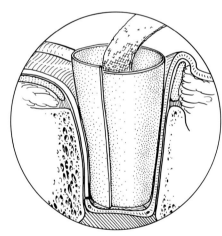

Figure 3-49

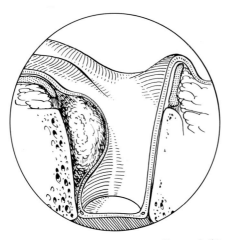

Figure 3-50

PROBLEMS AND SOLUTIONS

DISPLACED KÖRNER'S FLAP

This results from improper replacement of the Körner's flap at the end of the initial surgery. This can be prevented by careful replacement of the flap under microscopic observation and proper packing.

In a displaced Körner's flap, a fibrous mass may obstruct the posterolateral portion of the ear canal (Figure 3-50).

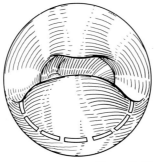

Figure 3-51

The entire obstructing mass is excised (Figure 3-51).

The exposed bone is covered by a postauricular full-thickness skin graft (Figure 3-52).

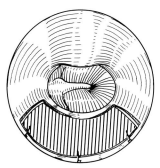

Figure 3-52

The canal is then packed (Figure 3-53). An alternative approach would be to create a medially based posterior canal flap by removing the fibrous tissues from the skin and replacing it against the posterior canal wall.

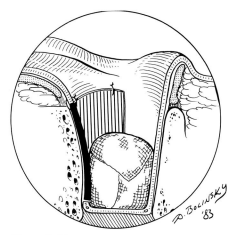

Figure 3-53

STENOSIS OF THE EAR CANAL

This can result from inadequate packing, early removal of the packing, postoperative infections, or improper placement of the skin grafts.

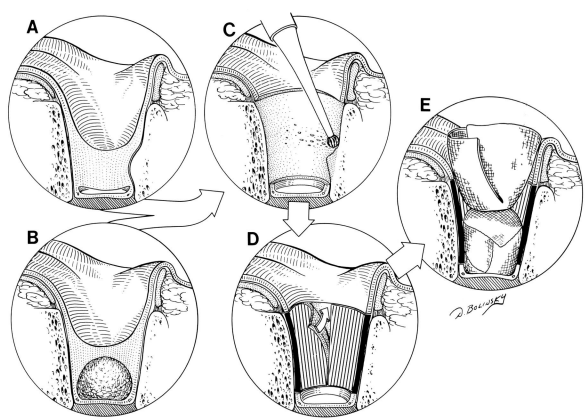

Figure 3-54

In ear canal stenosis, a fibrous mass may obstruct the entire bony portion of the ear canal (Figure 3-54A), or a rather thick, fibrous band may obstruct the midportions of the ear canal (Figure 3-54B). This is often associated with a cholesteatoma between this fibrous band and the tympanic membrane. The entire fibrous mass is excised, and the bony ear canal is widened to its maximum (Figure 3-54C). The exposed bony ear canal is entirely covered with a thin, full-thickness skin graft (Figure 3-54D), and the canal is packed (Figure 3-54E).

EROSION OF THE POSTERIOR BONY CANAL

This results from "extensive" thinning of the posterior bony canal at the time of the initial surgery or postoperative infection following the displacement of free or pedicle graft.

The erosion of the bone may or may not be connected with the mastoidectomy cavity (Figure 3-55). Cholesteatoma may coexist. The eroded bone is removed and a shallow, clean defect may be repaired by bone plug (or bone dust) and fascia.

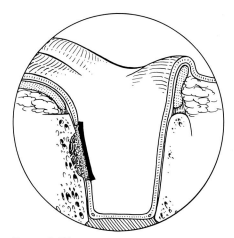

Figure 3-55

When the erosion is large and associated with either osteitis or deep cholesteatoma formation, a modified radical mastoidectomy with removal of the posterior canal wall is indicated (Figure 3-56).

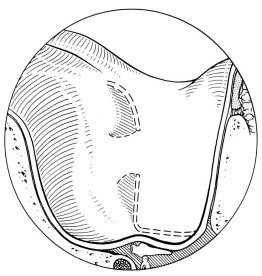

Figure 3-56

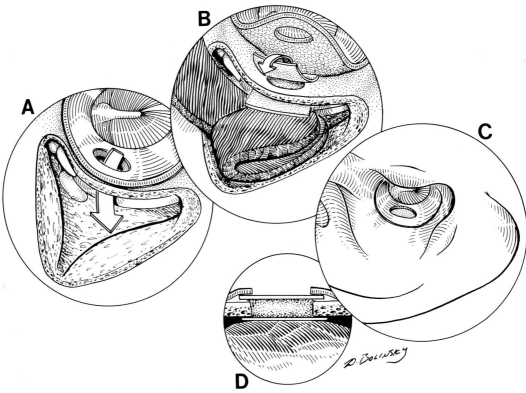

Figure 3-57

When the eroded area is limited but communicates with the mastoidectomy cavity, a postauricular simple mastoidectomy is first performed. The diseased bone is drilled or curetted away (Figure 3-57A). The bony canal wall is reconstructed by placing a bony or cartilaginous plug in the bony defect of the canal wall (Figure 3-57B), placing a fascia graft on both sides of the bony canal (Figure 3-57C) and a muscle-pedicled graft in the mastoidectomy cavity (Figure 3-57D). The elevated posterior canal skin is replaced, and the ear is packed.

REFERENCES

1. Chandler, J. R.: Malignant External Otitis. *Laryngoscope,* 78:1257–1294, 1968.
2. Chandler, J.: Pathogenesis and Treatment of Facial Paralysis Due to Malignant External Otitis. *Ann. Otol. Rhin. Laryngol.,* 81:648–658, 1972.
3. DiBartolomeo, J. R.: Exostosis of the External Auditory Canal. *Ann. Otol. Rhin. Laryngol.* (suppl. 61), 1979.
4. Graham, M. D.: Osteomas and Exostoses of the External Auditory Canal. A Clinical, Histopathologic and Scanning Electron Microscope Study. *Laryngoscope* 88:566–572, 1979.
5. Paparella, M. M.: Surgical Treatment of Intractable External otitis. *Laryngoscope,* 76:1138–1147, 1968.
6. Saunders, W. H. and Paparella, M. M.: Atlas of Ear Surgery, 2nd ed., Mosby, St. Louis, 1971.
7. Sheehy, J. L.: Osteoma of the External Auditory Canal. *Laryngoscope,* 68:1667–1673, 1958.
8. Sheehy, J. L.: Diffuse Exostoses and Osteomata of the External Auditory Canal: A Report of 100 Operations. *Otolaryngol. Head Neck Surg.,* 90:337–342, 1982.

4

Tympanoplasty Classification

Wullstein[5] classified tympanoplasty into five types; this classification is shown in modified form in Table 4-1.

Table 4-1
Classification of Tympanoplasty by Wullstein

Type	Damage to Middle Ear	Method of Repair
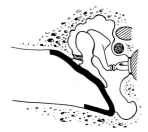		
I	Perforated Tympanic Membrane with Normal Ossicular Chain	Closure of Perforation Type I, Same as Myringoplasty

Table 4-1 (continued)

Type	Damage to Middle Ear	Method of Repair

| II | Perforation of Tympanic Membrane with Erosion of Malleus | Closure with Graft Against Incus or Remains of Malleus |

| III | Destruction of Tympanic Membrane and Ossicular Chain but with Intact and Mobile Stapes | Graft Contacts Normal Stapes; Also Gives Sound Protection for Round Window |

| IV | Similar to Type III, but Head, Neck, and Crura of Stapes Missing; Footplate Mobile | Mobile Footplate Left Exposed or Graft Attaches to Mobile Footplate; Air Pocket Between Round Window and Graft Provides Sound Protection for Round Window |

Va   Vb   Doolinsky '83

| V | Similar to Type IV Plus Fixed Footplate | Fenestra in Horizontal Semicircular Canal; Graft Seals off Middle Ear to Give Sound Protection for Round Window |

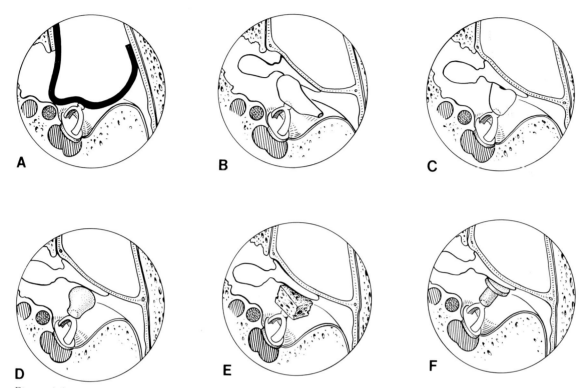

Figure 4-1

Farrior[2] proposed the following type of tympano-plasty according to the basic pathologic anatomy at the completion of the surgery, rather than classifying them according to the method of reconstruction utilized:

- Type I: Reconstruction of a new eardrum, intact malleus, incus, and stapes
- Type II: Reconstruction of a new eardrum in its natural position
- Type III: Reconstruction of a new eardrum on top of upright, freely mobile stapes
  —Type III: Classic (Figure 4-1A)
  —Type III IG: Incus graft (Figure 4-1B)
  —Type III IGM: Incus graft to malleus (Figure 4-1C)
  —Type III MG: Malleus head graft (Figure 4-1D)
  —Type III BG: Bone graft (Figure 4-1E)
  —Type III PORP: Partial ossicular replacement prosthesis (Figure 4-1F)

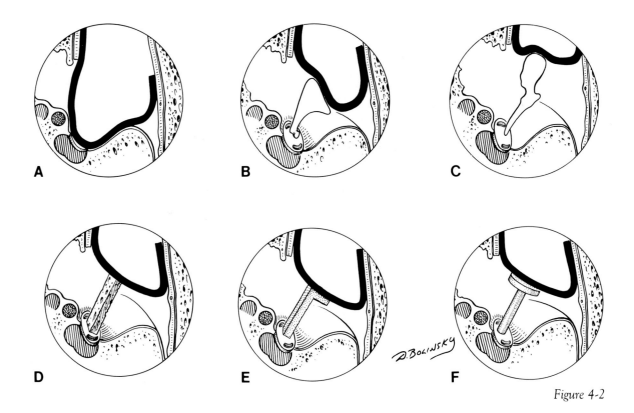

Figure 4-2

- Type IV: Reconstruction of a new eardrum and columella on footplate of stapes
  —Type IV: Classic (Figure 4-2A)
  —Type IV IG: Incus graft (Figure 4-2B)
  —Type IV MG: Malleus graft (Figure 4-2C)
  —Type IV BG: Bone graft (Figure 4-2D)
  —Type IV CG: Cartilage graft (Figure 4-2E)
  —Type IV TORP: Total ossicular replacement prosthesis (Figure 4-2F)
- Type V: Reconstruction of an eardrum either over a fistula in the horizontal semicircular canal or a new eardrum with a secondary fenestration of the horizontal semicircular canal

Saunders and Paparella modified Type V tympanoplasty (see Table 4-1), subdividing it into:

- Type Va: Fenestration of the horizontal semicircular canal
- Type Vb: Stapedectomy in cases of tympanoplasty Type IV with stapes fixation[3]

The best results in tympanoplasty are obtained when the stapes is upright and freely mobile regardless of the type of reconstruction utilized. In classifying tympanoplasty according to basic pathologic anatomy, all cases with intact stapedial superstructures are classified under Type III with indication of the type of superstructure by initials, as IG incus graft.[2]

REFERENCES

1. The Committee on Construction of Hearing of the American Academy of Ophthalmology and Otolaryngology: Standard Classification for Surgery of Chronic Ear Infection. *Arch. Otolaryngol.*, 81: 204–205, 1965.
2. Farrior, J. B.: Classification of Tympanoplasty. *Arch. Otolaryngol.*, 93:548–550, 1971.
3. Gacek, R. R.: Results of Modified Type V Tympanoplasty. *Laryngoscope,* 83:437–447, 1973.
4. Saunders, W. H., and Paparella, M. M.: Atlas of Ear Surgery, 2nd ed., Mosby, St. Louis, 1971.
5. Wullstein, H.: Funktionelle Operationen im Mittelohr mit Hilfe des freien Spaltlappen-Transplantates. *Arch. Ohren. Nasen. u. Kehlkopfh.,* 161:422, 1952.

5

—Myringoplasty—

The term "myringoplasty" is reserved for the simple repair of a tympanic membrane when no ossicular reconstruction is involved.

SELECTION OF APPROACHES

A tympanic membrane grafting can be accomplished by either a transcanal (endaural) or a postauricular approach. A transcanal repair can be done via a tympanic membrane perforation or a tympanotomy (Table 5-1).

Indications for a transcanal approach include a small perforation (less than 20 percent of the pars tensa of the tympanic membrane), medium-sized posterior perforation, wide ear canal with good visibility of the anterior border of the perforation, and no need for mastoidectomy.

Indications for a postauricular approach include narrow ear canal with poor visibility of anterior margins of the perforation, medium-to-large-sized anterior and inferior perforations, total perforation with or without absence of anterior annular tympanicus, and need for mastoidectomy.

Two basic grafting techniques are overlay or lateral grafting and underlay or medial grafting techniques. Following lateral grafting of the fascia, there appears to be higher incidence of postoperative complications such as lateral displacement of the graft, blunting of the anterior sulcus, canal stenosis, and inclusion cholesteatoma; hence the author now favors the medial grafting technique. Suggested approaches for various types of tympanic membrane perforation are shown in Figure 5-1.

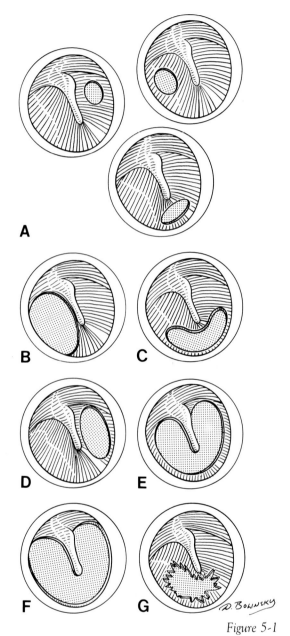

A

B   C

D   E

F   G

Figure 5-1

Table 5-1
Selection of Approaches

Perforation Loci	Approaches
Small perforations (<20% of Pars Tensa) (Figure 5-1A)	Transcanal Transtympanic Transcanal Tympanotomy
Posterior (Pars Tensa) Defect (Figure 5-1B)	Transcanal Tympanotomy Postauricular Tympanotomy
Inferior (Pars Tensa) Defect (Figure 5-1C)	Postauricular Tympanotomy
Anterior (Pars Tensa) Defect (Figure 5-1D)	Postauricular Tympanotomy
Total (Pars Tensa) Defect (Annulus Intact) (Figure 5-1E)	Postauricular Tympanotomy
Total (Pars Tensa) Defect (Annulus Absent) (Figure 5-1F)	Postauricular Tympanotomy Postauricular Tympanic Membrane Transplant
Traumatic Perforation (Figure 5-1G)	Transcanal Transtympanic Transcanal Tympanotomy

TYPES OF GRAFTS

Autogenous tissues of many types have been employed for the repair of tympanic membrane defects. Preference for one material over another has reflected the success or failure of any given graft in the hands of experienced otologists. Fundamental, however, to the success of any graft is the careful, nontraumatic harvesting and preservation of the material complemented by the meticulous placement of the graft.

Skin (split-thickness or full-thickness grafts)[17] may be readily obtained from a non-hair-bearing area of the forearm, thigh, or lower abdomen. A safety razor blade (free hand) or any one of several commercially available dermatomes may be used for the harvest (Figure 5-2A). Skin may be obtained from the postauricular region with no cosmetic insult (Figure 5-2B). Posterior canal wall skin has been

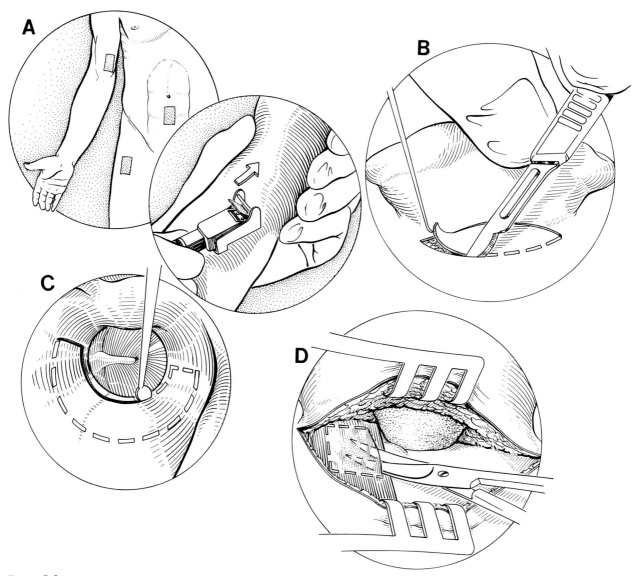

Figure 5-2

employed (Figure 5-2C).[7,8,12] Temporalis fascia[5,12,14] is currently the most widely used and most dependable material for tympanic membrane grafting (Figure 5-2D). The graft may be used in a moistened or dried state with equal success. The author dries the fascia first and moistens it immediately before its use. Some otologists make use of the thin areolar tissue that lies above the fascia—the so-called "fool's fascia."[3]

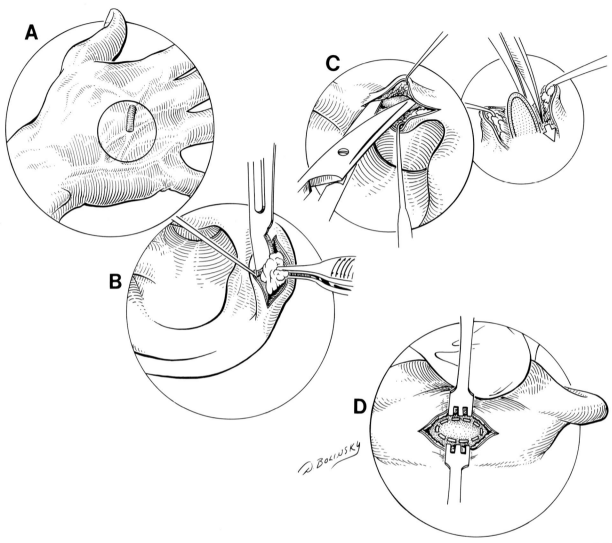

Figure 5-3

Vein from the dorsum of the hand has been successfully employed (Figure 5-3A).[11,15] Lobular fat is readily accessible and can be easily employed, especially in cases of those that lend themselves for office or clinical closure (Figure 5-3B).[10] Tragal perichondrium has proved to be an excellent autogenous graft material. Readily available in the field, the loss of the tragus leaves an acceptable cosmetic defect. Sharp scissor or knife dissection with fine hook retraction permit rapid delivery of the cartilage. The perichondrium may be stripped off on the back table or removed without excising the tragus if the surgeon does not wish to remove the cartilage (Figure 5-3C).[4] The conchal cartilage is another potential source for perichondrium that is readily available in the operating field (Figure 5-3D).[16]

SURGICAL TECHNIQUES

TRANSCANAL TRANSTYMPANIC APPROACH

The perforation should be clearly visualized following the evacuation of ceruminous material and squamous debris from the canal (Figure 5-4). The speculum holder should be placed to afford optimal visualization and positional maneuverability for the surgeon.

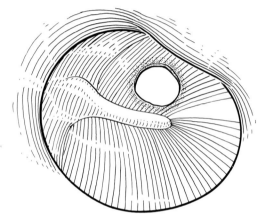

Figure 5-4

A 2–3-mm right-angle hook scores the medial surface of the membrane around the perforation (Figure 5-5A). Note the careful underscoring of the drum over the manubrium; this is highlighted in Figure 5-5B.

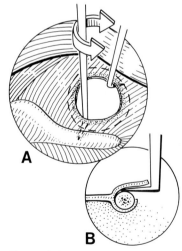

Figure 5-5

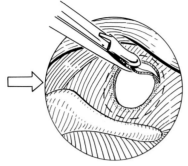

Figure 5-6

The sickle knife is pushed through all three layers of the tympanic membrane at one point, and the circumferential incision is made by up-and-down movements around the edge of the perforation; the fibrous rim of the perforation is then carefully removed with a cup forceps (Figure 5-6).

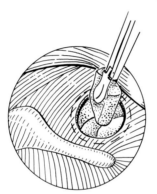

Figure 5-7

Gelfoam impregnated with antibiotic solution is placed in the middle-ear space (Figure 5-7).

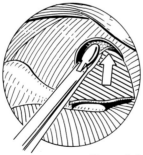

Figure 5-8

The graft is inserted into the middle ear: a Derlacki mobilizer, a sickle knife, or another fine instrument delivers the graft while a Billeau wax loop permits the anterior placement of the graft atraumatically (Figure 5-8).

The graft is laid flush against the manubrium or in the space between the manubrium and the tympanic membrane placed evenly under the perforation (Figure 5-9).

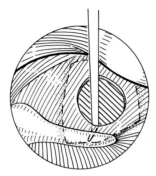

Figure 5-9

A separate small piece of fascia may be placed lateral to the perforation. Gelfoam is juxtaposed laterally, and the canal is packed (Figure 5-10).

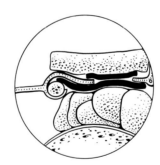

Figure 5-10

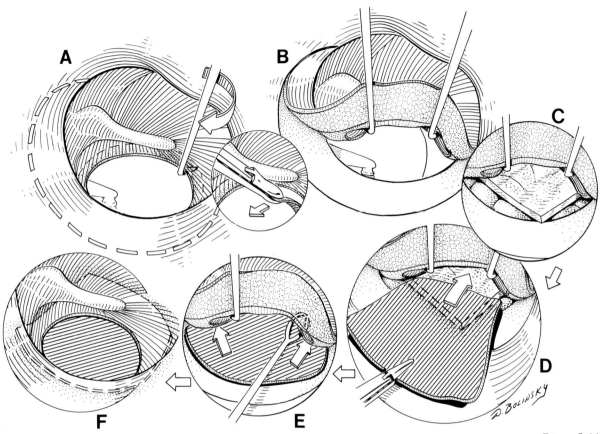

Figure 5-11

TRANSCANAL TYMPANOTOMY APPROACH

The margins of the perforation are scored and freshened as previously described (Figure 5-11). The tympanomeatal flap is elevated 5–6 mm from the annulus from the 12 o'clock to 6 o'clock position. The insert to Figure 5-11A shows the removal of a freshened rim from the circumference of the perforation. To remove the scored rim, it is necessary to incise the edges of the perforation first with the sickle knife while the remnant of the tympanic membrane is still under tension. The tympanic membrane is elevated with preservation of the fibrous annulus and the denuding of the undersurface of the perforation completed (Figure 5-11B).

Gelfoam is placed in the middle ear. A sheet of Gelfilm serves as a guide on which the graft may be "slid" into the middle ear (Figure 5-11C). The graft is introduced and positioned (Figure 5-11D).

Care is exercised in ensuring that the graft lies flat against the denuded portion of the membrane, especially anteriorly (Figure 5-11E). Placement of additional Gelfoam in the middle ear space at this time will help bring the graft up against the tympanic membrane. The tympanomeatal flap is replaced (Figure 5-11F). Care is taken to ensure that the edges of the flap are not inverted to prevent postoperative cholesteatoma formation. The canal is then packed.

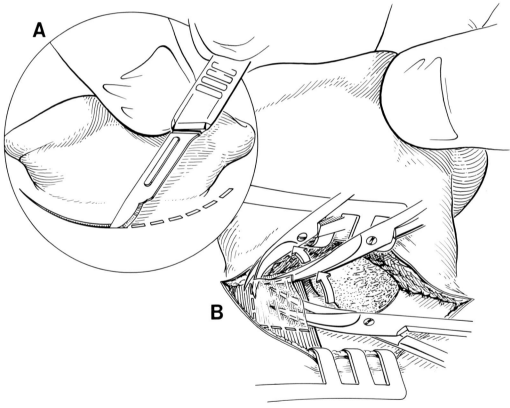

Figure 5-12

POSTAURICULAR TYMPANOTOMY APPROACH

A standard postauricular incision is made several millimeters posterior to the auricular crease (Figure 5-12A). Temporalis fascia is harvested for grafting (Figure 5-12B).

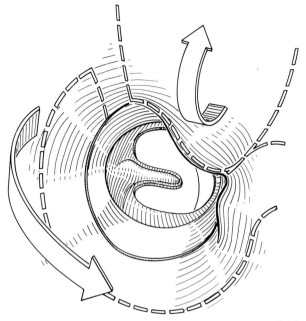

The auricle is retracted forward and the canal entered at the level of the mastoid cortex. Canal incisions are made at 12 o'clock and 6 o'clock and joined medially at 3–5 mm from the annulus. An anterior canal wall flap is elevated from medial to lateral. The posterior canal wall skin is elevated as an inferolaterally pedicled flap. (Figure 5-13.)

Figure 5-13

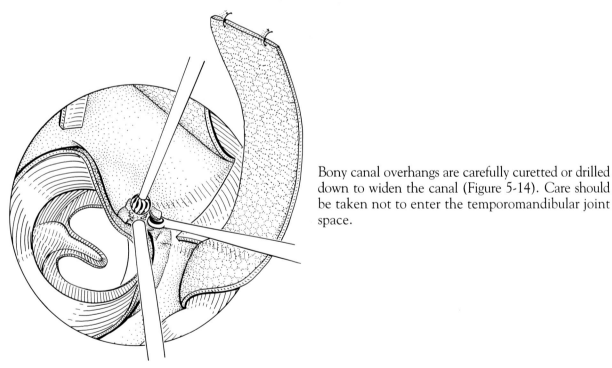

Bony canal overhangs are carefully curetted or drilled down to widen the canal (Figure 5-14). Care should be taken not to enter the temporomandibular joint space.

Figure 5-14

If the anterior bony bulge (artist's view shown in Figure 5-15) is not removed, blunting of the graft at the anterior sulcus may result.

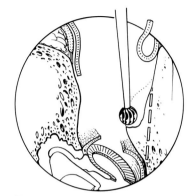

Figure 5-15

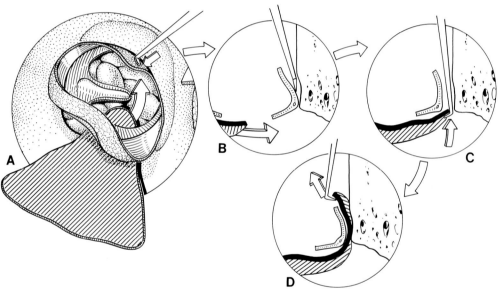

Figure 5-16

The margins of the perforation are denuded and epithelial remnants are cleaned away. The middle ear is packed with antibiotic impregnated Gelfoam and the fibrous annulus carefully elevated. The graft is introduced (Figure 5-16A). Figure 5-16B–D shows the placement of the graft against the anterior sulcus. Note that an anterior edge of the graft is brought out into the canal through a small slit made between the annulus and the bony sulcus. This will prevent the medial displacement of the graft.

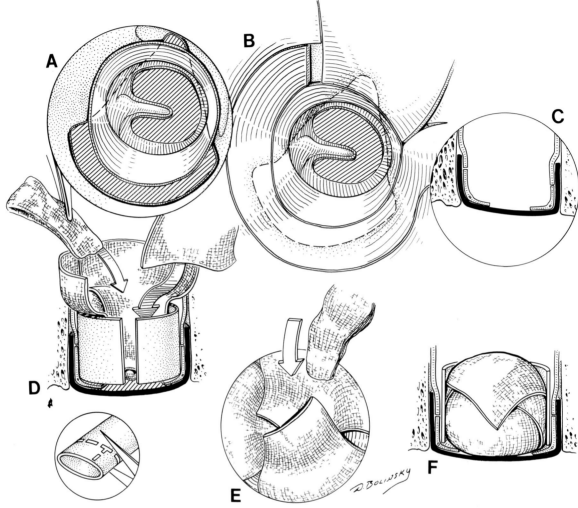

Figure 5-17

The graft is placed so that it extends over the lip of the anterior bony annulus as well as draping the posterior wall (Figure 5-17A). The inferolaterally based skin pedicle is placed down on the bony canal wall posteriorly while the anterior skin flap is replaced (Figure 5-17B). A cross section showing the position of the graft is illustrated in Figure 5-17C. The ear canal is packed using a double-pack technique (Figure 5-17D–F). Note that the medial pack consisting of three strips of surgical rayon and petrolatum (Vaseline) gauze is placed medial to the ½-inch rubber drain. This will ensure an easy atraumatic removal of the packing.

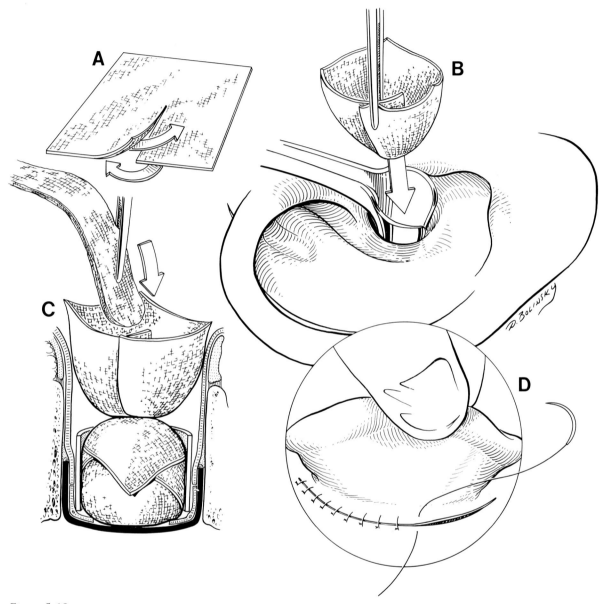

Figure 5-18

The outer pack consists of an Owen's gauze sleeve and antibiotic impregnated ½-inch Vaseline gauze (Figure 5-18A–D).

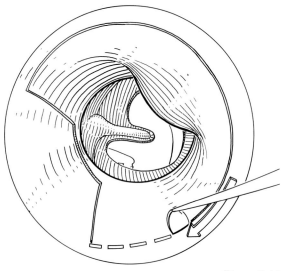

Figure 5-19

ALTERNATIVE PROCEDURES

Sheehy's Lateral (Overlay) Graft Technique[12]

Superiorly, an incision is made in the tympano-squamous suture line while a posterior incision is made in the tympanomastoid suture line (Figure 5-19). These are connected by a semicircular incision approximately 1–2 mm from the annulus. The vascular strip is thus preserved. A circumferential incision is made slightly external to the junction of the outer and middle thirds of the canal, connecting the two suture line incisions.

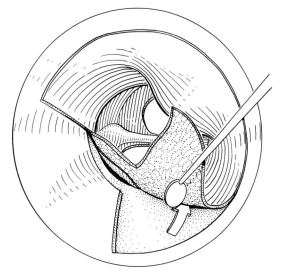

Elevation is carried medially to the annulus, which is not disturbed (Figure 5-20). The canal skin and remnant of deepithelized layer are raised as one piece. When the flap is completely elevated, it is removed and preserved.

Figure 5-20

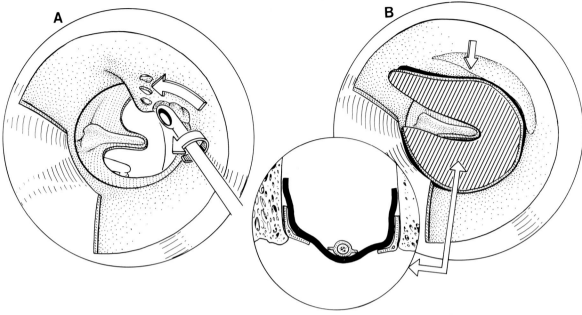

Figure 5-21

With drill or curet, all bony overhangs are reduced
and the canal maximally widened (Figure 5-21A).
The mastoid air cell system should not be entered,
however. Careful inspection under magnification
should be carried out to ensure that all the squamous layer of the tympanic membrane has been
removed. The rehydrated fascia graft is placed external to the denuded tympanic membrane (Figure
5-21B). A Billeau ear loop is used to adapt it to
the remnant. The graft is notched to slip about the
manubrium.

The anterior graft of the fascia is turned back over
the exposed manubrium. (Figure 5-22).

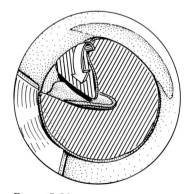

Figure 5-22

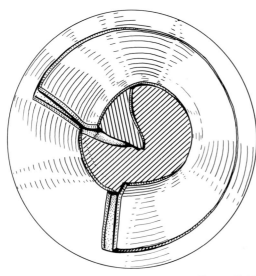

The skin graft is returned (Figure 5-23). Care should be employed especially anteriorly where blunting may occur. Note a lip of skin overlying the fascia graft by a few millimeters in Figure 5-23.

SOOY PEDICLED GRAFT TECHNIQUE

As in all myringoplastic procedures, the margins of the perforation are denuded and the freshened edges scored. A posterosuperiorly based canal skin flap is raised (approximate size 1 × 3 cm) (Figure 5-24A).

Superficial epithelium is removed from the margins of the perforation, and an autogenous (vein) graft is placed over a bed of antibiotic impregnated Gelfoam (Figure 5-24B). The pedicle is placed over the graft, and the canal is packed after placing a thin paper patch over the pedicle (Figure 5-24C).

Figure 5-23

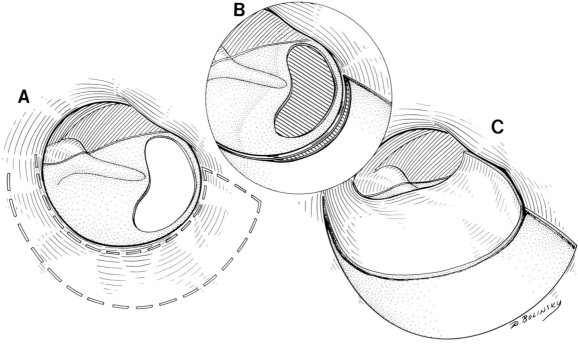

Figure 5-24

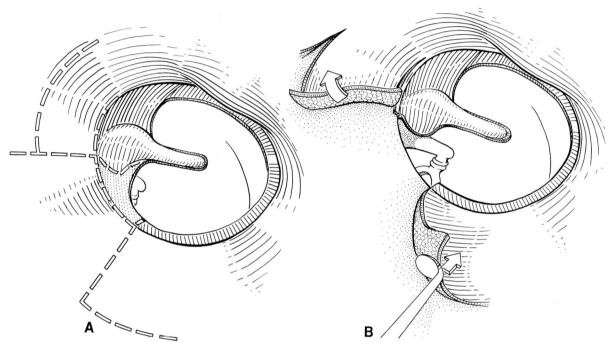

Figure 5-25

GLASSCOCK UNDERLAY TECHNIQUE

A total perforation (annulus intact) is depicted in Figure 5-25A. A vascular strip is defined by incisions along the tympanosquamous and tympanomastoid suture lines. The vascular strip is retracted out of the field of elevation by a retractor while an inferior flap is elevated down to the annulus (Figure 5-25B). All anterior bony overhangs are removed as optimal vision of the field is obtained.

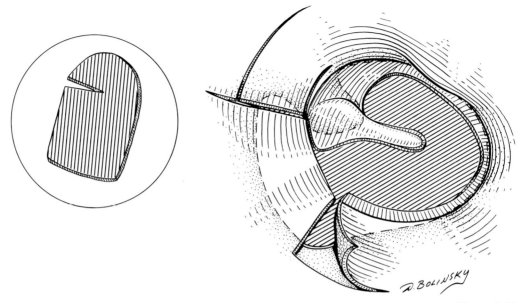

Figure 5-26

The notched (for the malleus) fascia graft (Figure 5-26 insert) is introduced medial to the annulus by a cup forceps (Figure 5-26). Prior to this the middle ear is packed with antibiotic impregnated Gelfoam. A fine-needle suction and sickle knife may be used to position the graft. The graft drapes the posterior canal wall. The canal wall skin and inferior annulus are repositioned.

FISCH UNDERLAY TECHNIQUE

Canal wall flaps are elevated several millimeters from the annulus (Figure 5-27A). The superior and inferior flaps are elevated independently to the annulus.

The margins of the perforation are denuded and the middle ear packed (Figure 5-27B). The notched graft is placed and directed under the anterior and posterior rims of the fibrous annulus. The graft drapes the posterior canal wall. Note that the notched graft (shown in Figure 5-27B) is placed around the manubrium and the umbo is lateral to the graft. This will prevent lateralization and will maintain the cone shape of the grafted membrane. The canal flaps are returned and the canal is packed (Figure 5-27C).

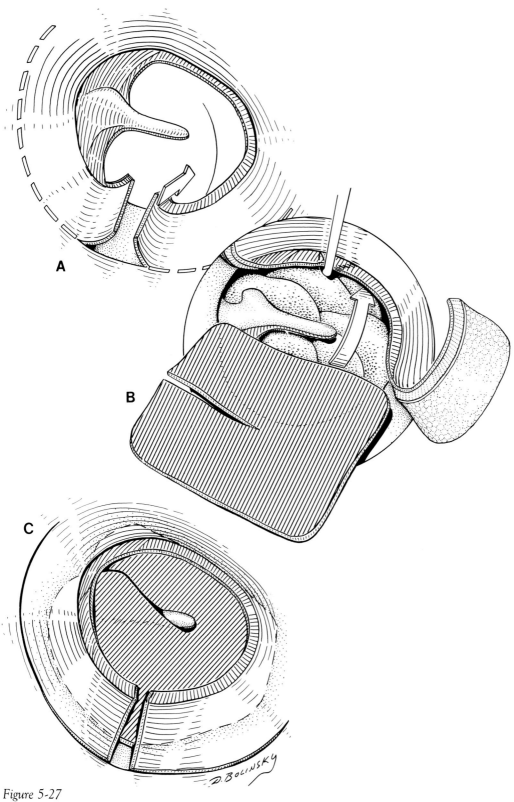

A

B

C

D. BOLINSKY

Figure 5-27

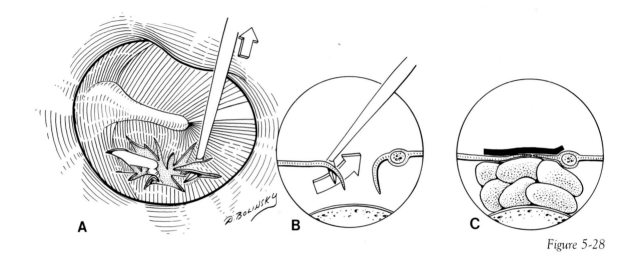

A   B   C

Figure 5-28

GELFOAM MYRINGOPLASTY TECHNIQUE

This procedure is for immediate repair of a post-traumatic perforation. Following the scrupulous cleansing of the canal, the fine margins of the perforation are exteriorized from the perforation (Figure 5-28A).

A 3-mm hook may be used to elevate all the drum tears from the middle-ear space (Figure 5-28B). This step is of paramount importance in prevention of development of a cholesteatoma. Antibiotic-soaked Gelfoam is placed in the middle-ear space (Figure 5-28C). A Gelfoam plaque is placed lateral to this. The canal is packed.

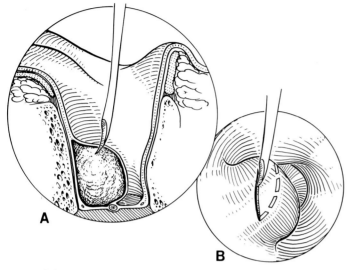

Figure 5-29

PROBLEMS AND SOLUTIONS

CANAL WALL INCLUSION CHOLESTEATOMA

Posterior canal wall cholesteatomatous mass is perforated by gentle pressure with a sickle knife (Figure 5-29A). The walls are incised in an ellipse (Figure 5-29B).

The contents are spooned out and suctioned by use of a round or oval knife (Figure 5-30).

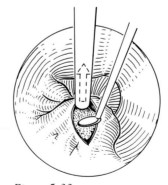

Figure 5-30

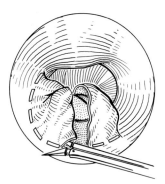

Figure 5-31

Posterior canal wall skin is excised including the sac covering (Figure 5-31).

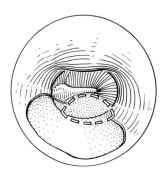

Figure 5-32

The excision is carried medially and anteriorly, including a portion of the tympanic drum membrane (Figure 5-32).

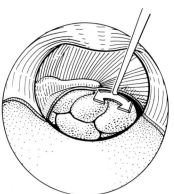

Figure 5-33

The margins of the perforation are freshened and packing placed in the middle ear (Figure 5-33).

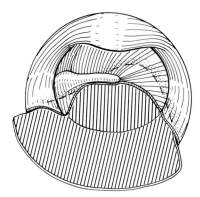

The temporalis fascia graft is placed medial to the margins of the perforation, and extends posteriorly onto the bony wall (Figure 5-34).

Figure 5-34

RETRACTION AND MIDDLE-EAR EFFUSION

Retraction pockets may develop when the Eustachian tube is malfunctioning and may become a cause of postoperative cholesteatoma and persistent hearing loss (Figure 5-35).

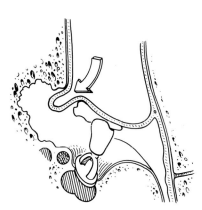

Figure 5-35

After the posterior canal wall skin has been elevated, the retracted membranes are removed and a graft placed against the cartilage or bone graft in the attic (Figure 5-36). It is placed medial to the canal skin and the malleus.

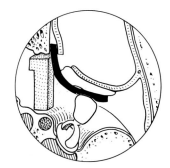

Figure 5-36

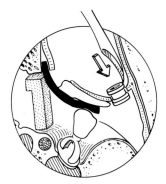

Figure 5-37

A tympanotomy ventilation tube may temporarily permit optimal aeration of the tympanic cavity as the graft heals and prevent negative pressure that contributes to graft retraction (Figure 5-37).

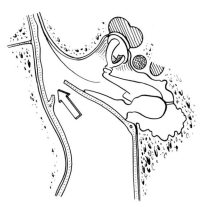
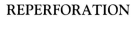

Figure 5-38

REPERFORATION

Reperforation, especially along the margin of the anterior sulcus, is a major problem (Figure 5-38). Often this follows a medial graft technique and is due to failure to smooth out the curvature of the bony wall before grafting and inadequate placement of the anterior portions of the graft.

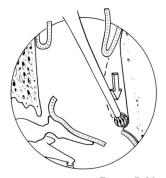

Figure 5-39

Canal flaps are elevated and the bony anterior sulcus is taken down, creating a "bony" shelf (Figure 5-39).

A medial graft is placed (Figure 5-40). Note that the anterior edge of the fascia graft is placed over (lateral to) the newly created bony shelf.

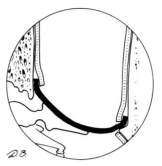

Figure 5-40

ANTERIOR BLUNTING

The tympanic membrane graft is noted to have become blunted along the anterior sulcus (Figure 5-41). Fibrous tissue is seen to have filled in the space. Furthermore, note the bulge in the bony anterior canal wall.

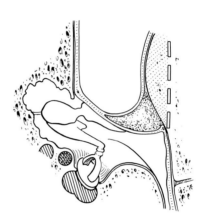

Figure 5-41

Canal wall flaps are elevated (Figure 5-42A) following incisions as described in Figure 5-13. A circumferential rim of tissue is raised 2 mm from the annulus.

The bony anterior canal wall is reduced and a graft is placed lateral to the defect (Figure 5-42B). An additional skin graft may be required to prevent recurrent blunting.

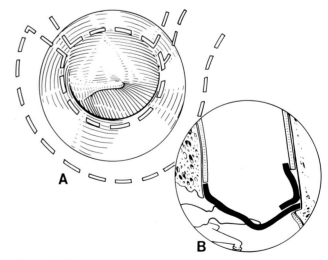

Figure 5-42

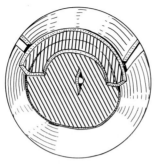

Figure 5-43

The flaps are returned with the umbo piercing the fascia graft (Figure 5-43). Note further that the graft extends onto the posterior canal wall.

An alternative technique that may be employed in the restoration of the air conducting mechanism in this case would be the employment of a homograft tympanic membrane.

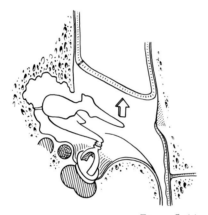

Figure 5-44

LATERALIZATION

The tympanic membrane graft has lateralized and completely separated from the ossicular chain (Figure 5-44). Note the small bony edge anteriorly.

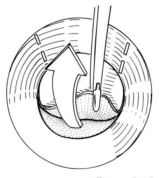

Figure 5-45

Independent skin flaps posteriorly and anteriorly are elevated (Figure 5-45). The graft is elevated, exposing the middle ear, and removed.

All bony canal wall irregularities are reduced (Figure 5-46).

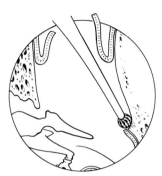

Figure 5-46

A lateral graft is placed (Figure 5-47). Note the smooth even placement of the canal skin flaps applied over the graft.

Alternatively, as described in Figure 5-47, a homograft tympanic membrane may be employed in the reconstruction of the sound-conducting mechanism in this case.

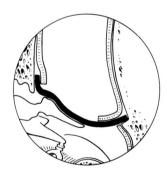

Figure 5-47

REFERENCES

1. Farrior, J. B.: Incisions in Tympanoplasty; Anatomic Considerations and Indications. *Laryngoscope,* 93:75–86, 1983.
2. Fisch, U.: Tympanoplasty and Stapedectomy—A Manual of Technique. Georg Thieme Verlag, Stuttgart, 1980.
3. Glasscock, M. E.: Tympanic Membrane Grafting with Fascia: Overlay vs. Undersurface Technique. *Laryngoscope,* 83:754–770, 1973.
4. Goodhill, V.: Tragal Perichondrium and Cartilage in Tympanoplasty. *Arch Otolaryngol.,* 85:480–491, 1967.
5. Herrmann, A.: Trommelfellplastik mit Fasciengewebe vom Musculus temporalis nach Begradiung der vorderen Gehörgangswand, *HNO* (Berl.), 9:136, 1961.
6. Hough, J. V. D.: Tympanoplasty with the Interior Fascial Graft Technique and Ossicular Reconstruction. *Laryngoscope,* 80:1385–1413, 1970.
7. House, W. F. and Sheehy, J. L.: Myringoplasty: use of ear canal skin compared with other techniques. *Arch. Otolaryngol.,* 73:407–415, 1961.
8. Plester, D.: Fortschritte in der Mikrochirurgie des Ohres in den letzten 10 Jahren. *HNO* (Berl.), 18:33, 1970.
9. Shambaugh, G. E., Jr. and Glasscock, M. E., III: Surgery of the Ear, 3rd ed., Saunders, Philadelphia, 1980.
10. Ringenberg, J. C. and Fornatto, E. J.: The Fat Graft in Middle Ear Surgery. *Arch. Otolaryngol.,* 76:407–412, 1962.
11. Shea, J. J.: Vein Graft Closure of Eardrum Perforations. *J. Laryng. Otol.,* 74:358, 1960.
12. Sheehy, J. L.: Surgery of Chronic Otitis Media. In: Otolaryngology, Vol. I, G. M. English (Ed.). Harper & Row, New York, chap. 20, pp. 1–87, 1977.
13. Sooy, F. A.: A Method of Repairing a Large Marginal Perforation. *Ann. Otol.,* 65:911, 1956.
14. Storrs, L. A.: Myringoplasty with the Use of Fascia Grafts. *Arch. Otolaryngol.,* 74:45–49, 1961.
15. Tabb, H. G.: Closure of Perforations of the Tympanic Membrane by Vein Grafts: A Preliminary Report of 20 Cases. *Laryngoscope,* 70:271, 1960.
16. Wiesel, J. M., Gay, I., and Wexler, M. R.: Conchal Perichondrium in Tympanoplasty. *Laryngoscope,* 90:1236–1237, 1980.
17. Wullstein, H.: Funktionelle Operationen im Mittelohr mit Hilfe des freien Spaltlappen-Transplantates. *Arch. Ohren-Nasen- u. Kehlkopfh.,* 161:422, 1952.

6

Ossicular Reconstruction

Creative procedures may be required to reestablish the air-conducting mechanism in those patients who have sustained fixation, dislocation, or dissolution of the ossicular chain as a result of trauma, infection, or iatrogenic removal of the ossicular mass or portions thereof in previous surgical procedures such as fenestration or mastoidectomy. A smaller but important patient subgroup would be those who have congenital problems affecting the ossicular mass.

GRAFT MATERIALS

Since a wide variety of potential reconstructive techniques may potentially be applied with each tympanoplastic procedure, the surgeon should be familiar with the commonly employed autograft, homograft, and xenograft materials available.

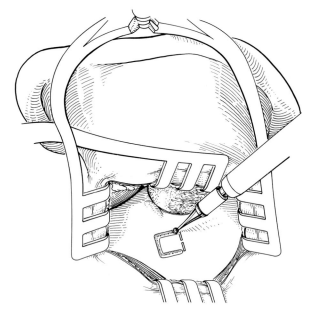

Figure 6-1

CORTICAL BONE

Bone from the cortex lying posterior and superior to the margins of the mastoid (or cavity) may be easily harvested (Figure 6-1). An outline of the autograft is made with a 1-mm chisel and subsequently the perimeter of the graft outline is burred.

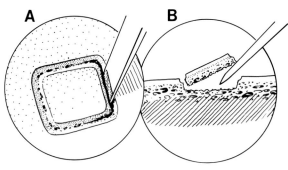

Figure 6-2

The margins of the graft are undermined with a broad flat 2–3-mm chisel (Figure 6-2A). The graft is elevated as one would open a trap door (Figure 6-2B). Care must be taken not to violate either an undisturbed mastoid or, more seriously, the posterior fossa.

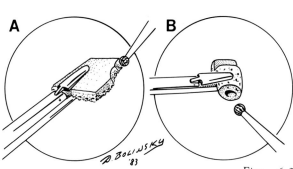

Figure 6-3

The graft is maintained in physiologic solution until it is time to shape it for placement (Figure 6-3A). When its final shape is defined, the graft should be held firmly and in a safe location (not over the operative field) to mitigate the possibility of losing the graft. The final graft design is demonstrated in Figure 6-3B. A small acetabulum has been bored out to fit the capitulum of the stapes.

TYMPANIC SPINE
(J. B. FARRIOR)

The anterior tympanic spine may be harvested for interposition grafting (Figure 6-4A). Figure 6-4B is a cross-sectional view of tympanic spine showing the fine chisel used to harvest this bone.

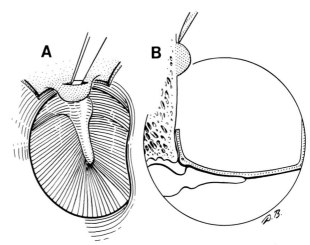

Figure 6-4

HOMOGRAFTS

Surgeons who perform a fair amount of ear surgery often establish their own "bank" for *homograft ossicles* (Figure 6-5). These bones may be used as anatomically defined or burred to fit a given situation.

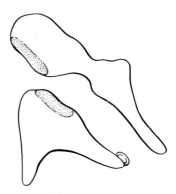

Figure 6-5

TORP AND PORP

In the last ten years, otologists worldwide have employed total ossicular replacement prostheses (TORP) and partial ossicular replacement prostheses (PORP) (Figure 6-6). Extrusion rates of 2–5 percent have been reported. Often extrusion occurs early and is frequently associated with the technique employed in placement.

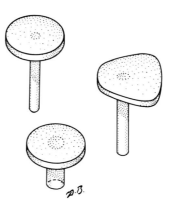

Figure 6-6

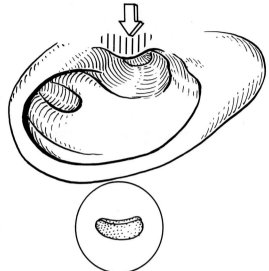

CARTILAGE

Because of its availability and stable metabolic characteristics, cartilage has been frequently employed (Figure 6-7). Here *tragal cartilage* is harvested. Note (in Figure 6-7) that the attendant mucoperichondrium on one side of the graft is left.

Figure 6-7

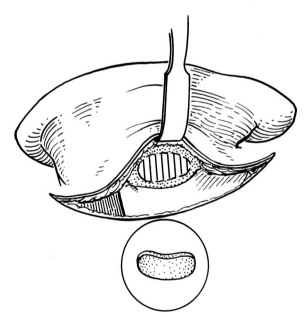

With a postauricular incision made for mastoid surgery, the surgeon need undermine only the auricular skin to obtain conchal cartilage (Figure 6-8). Alternatively, a separate incision may be made on the posterior portion of the auricle.

Figure 6-8

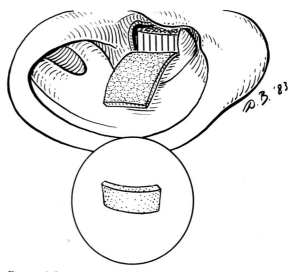

Often discarded, the conchal cartilage that is separated from the posterior canal skin when performing a Körner's flap may be just the size of cartilage needed for a graft (Figure 6-9).

Figure 6-9

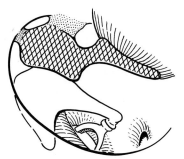

Figure 6-10

SURGICAL TECHNIQUES

MALLEUS PROBLEMS

Fixation

Anterior and superior malleolar fixation is noted (Figure 6-10).

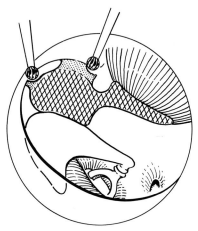

Figure 6-11

Careful burring of the bony and fibrous portions that are fixed is performed following satisfactory exposure through an atticotomy (Figure 6-11). Surgeons should be aware that vibratory trauma to the stapes footplate may occur if ossicular continuity is present.

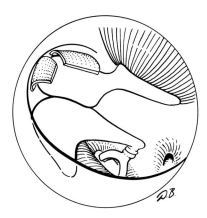

Figure 6-12

Silastic sheeting is juxtaposed on the raw bony surface that has been burred down (Figure 6-12).

To obviate the problem noted in Figures 6-10 and 6-11, the incudostapedial joint is disarticulated prior to burring (Figure 6-13).

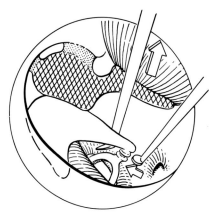

Figure 6-13

As shown in Figure 6-14, removal of the incus has been performed, and with the use of a malleus nipper, the head of the malleus is disarticulated carefully without traumatizing the drum.

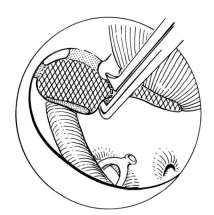

Figure 6-14

The head of the malleus is now shaped to fit between the capitulum of the stapes and manubrium of the malleus (Figure 6-15A). Figure 6-15B shows the sculptured malleus head in position. An artist's view in Figure 6-15C demonstrates the columella created by using the shaped malleus head.

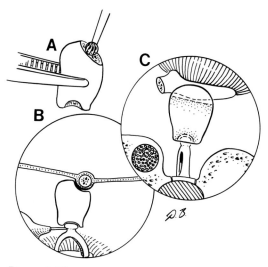

Figure 6-15

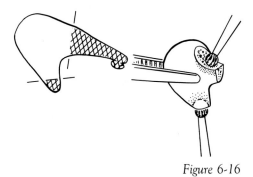

Figure 6-16

Following disarticulation and removal of the incus, the long process of the incus and its short process are removed and burred (Figure 6-16).

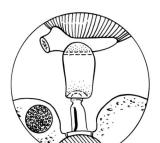
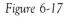

Figure 6-17

The contoured and sculptured incus rests between the stapes capitulum and the long process of the malleus (Figure 6-17).

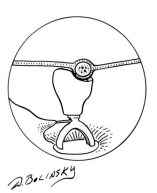

Figure 6-18

An artist's view demonstrates in Figure 6-18 the position of the sculptured incus.

Dislocation
(Incudomalleolar Separation)

Dislocation of the malleus may occur during surgical procedures or traumatic events. Figure 6-19 shows that the incus and malleus have separated within the confines of the epitympanic space.

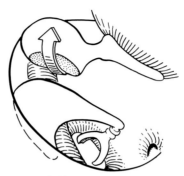

Figure 6-19

Figure 6-20 shows an incus rotated and juxtaposed on the stapes capitulum and manubrium of the malleus.

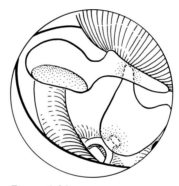

Figure 6-20

Figure 6-21 shows that the incus has been disarticulated and sculptured as demonstrated in Figures 6-16, 6-17, and 6-18 and placed in position on the stapes capitulum and manubrium of the malleus.

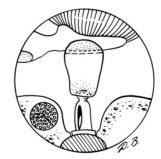

Figure 6-21

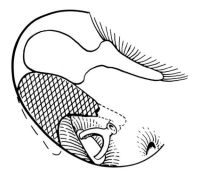

Figure 6-22

INCUS PROBLEMS

Necrosis

Figure 6-22 demonstrates a commonly found clinical problem due to chronic middle-ear-space infection. The lenticular process of the incus has necrosed. This is commonly due to the poor blood supply to this area.

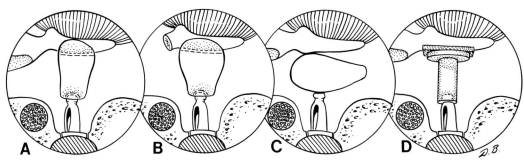

Figure 6-23

Restoration of ossicular continuity may be brought about by either using a sculptured incus homograft or the sculptured autograft (Figure 6-23A) disarticulating the head of the malleus and sculpturing it for placement as a columella (Figure 6-23B), employing an incus homograft or the autograft incus (Figure 6-23C), or using a PORP with a small piece of cartilage or autogenous tissue juxtaposed against the manubrium of the malleus (Figure 6-23D). Some surgeons place the head of the PORP partially against the malleus and partially against the tympanic membrane.

Dislocation

Figure 6-24 demonstrates dislocation of the lenticular process from the capitulum of the stapes. If technically feasible, reapproximation at this joint without stress would be an optimal restorative procedure; however, this is seldom possible.

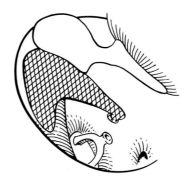

Figure 6-24

Figure 6-25 demonstrates the placement of a small piece of bone between the lenticular process of the incus and the capitulum of the stapes.

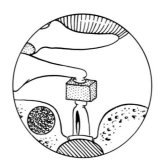

Figure 6-25

Figure 6-26 demonstrates a sculptured incus autograft being used to restore the conductive mechanism.

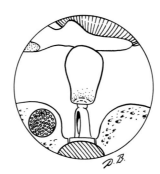

Figure 6-26

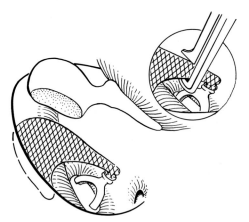

Figure 6-27 demonstrates the traumatic disruption of the incudomalleolar joint and epitympanic displacement of the incus. The surgeon must be careful when manipulating the incus to define the extent of dislocation with the suprastructure of the stapes if any exists. A small insert demonstrates the atraumatic severing of the long process of the incus, leaving it attached to the stapes capitulum.

Figure 6-27

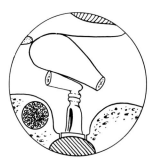

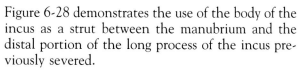

Figure 6-28 demonstrates the use of the body of the incus as a strut between the manubrium and the distal portion of the long process of the incus previously severed.

Figure 6-28

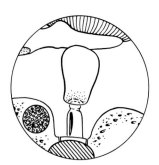

Figure 6-29 shows a sculptured incus columella.

Figure 6-29

Figure 6-30 demonstrates fibrous adhesion between the long process of the incus and the manubrium of the malleus, indicating that separation from the stapes suprastructure has occurred.

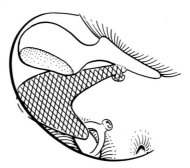

Figure 6-30

As shown in Figures 6-28 and 6-29, the body of the incus may be separated from its long process and used as a sandwich columella-type graft, or as shown in Figure 6-31 may be shaped as a sculptured incus graft.

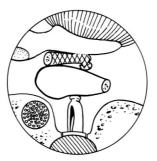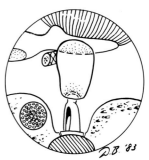

Figure 6-31

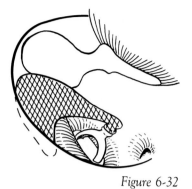

Figure 6-32

Fixation

Figure 6-32 demonstrates fixation of the incus. As previously mentioned, the reestablishment of a mobile ossicular chain is the goal of the ossiculoplasty.

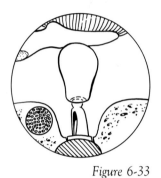

Figure 6-33

In Figure 6-33 a sculptured incus is placed between the manubrium and the capitulum of the stapes.

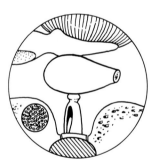

Figure 6-34

Figure 6-34 demonstrates the alternative positioning of the sculptured incus.

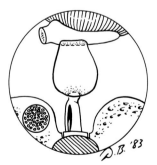

Figure 6-35

Figure 6-35 demonstrates the sculptured malleolar head grafted into place.

Absence

Absence of the incus is most commonly due to trauma or prior surgery (Figure 6-36).

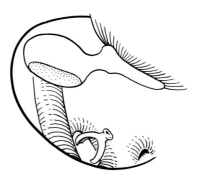

Figure 6-36

Following demonstration of a mobile stapes footplate, a sculptured malleolar head graft is placed (Figure 6-37). The insert in Figure 6-37 shows the amputation of the malleus head using the House-Dieter malleus nipper.

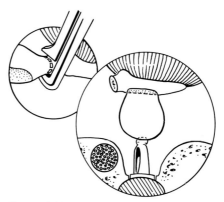

Figure 6-37

Alternatively, autogenous material such as cartilage may be employed to act as a strut (Figure 6-38).

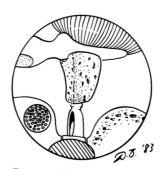

Figure 6-38

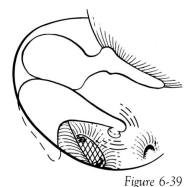

Figure 6-39

STAPES PROBLEMS

Absence

The stapes, like the malleus and incus, may be traumatized or subjected to fixation secondary to inflammation (Figure 6-30).

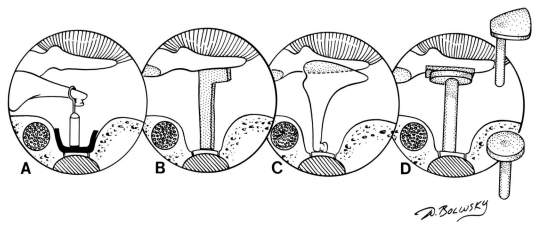

Figure 6-40

Following the satisfactory demonstration of a mobile footplate, an autogenous graft may be placed over the mobilized footplate or a piston may be placed (Figure 6-40A). Figure 6-40B demonstrates the placement of a cartilage columella, and Figure 6-40C demonstrates the placement of the autograft incus. Figure 6-40D demonstrates the placement of a TORP that may, as previously noted, juxtapose the manubrium of the malleus or partially juxtapose the malleus and the tympanic membrane. We recommend the placement of cartilage between the tympanic membrane and lateral portion of the TORP.

Fracture and Dislocation

Figure 6-41 demonstrates the fracture of the stapes cura.

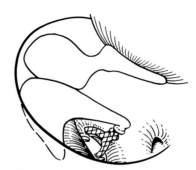

Figure 6-41

Figure 6-42 represents essentially an open reduction and fixation of the stapes suprastructure placed back in its anatomic position. Gelfoam is placed about the fracture site.

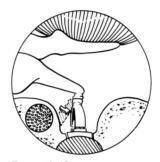

Figure 6-42

Figure 6-43 shows that the fractured stapes suprastructure has been removed and a House wire has been placed between the long process of the incus and the mobile footplate.

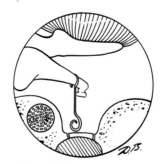

Figure 6-43

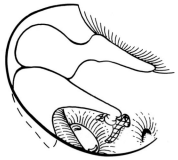

Figure 6-44

Figure 6-44 shows that the stapes suprastructure has been traumatically dislocated from the footplate region.

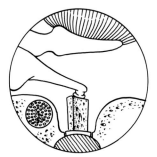

Figure 6-45

Figure 6-45 demonstrates the placement of autogenous cartilage over the mobile footplate from the lenticular process of the incus.

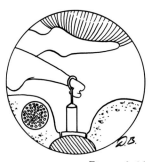

Figure 6-46

Figure 6-46 demonstrates the placement of a Teflon wire piston in traditional stapedotomy technique fashion.

The stapes suprastructure shown in Figure 6-47 has been disarticulated from the incus. It has been depressed into the oval window niche.

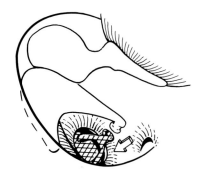

Figure 6-47

With careful placement of a right-angle hook between the crura of the stapes suprastructure, the stapes is gently mobilized from its depressed position within the oval window niche (Figure 6-48). The surgeon should be cognizant of the fact that any manipulation of the stapes within the confines of the vestibule may predispose to a sensorineural hearing loss and also that vigorous manipulation of the stapes with an angled hook may cause disruption of the incus.

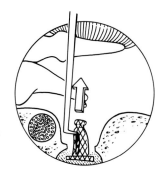

Figure 6-48

After the stapes has been repositioned, Gelfoam is placed about the suprastructure and footplate to prevent depression or aberrant positioning (Figure 6-49).

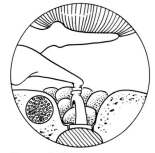

Figure 6-49

A fat-wire prosthesis is placed following the removal of the stapes in case repositioning of the stapes is not feasible (Figure 6-50).

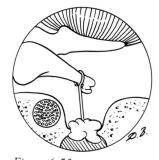

Figure 6-50

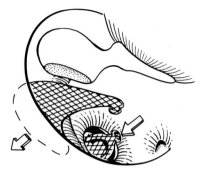

Figure 6-51

Figure 6-51 shows concomitant disruption of the incudostapedial joint with depression of the stapes and epitympanic recession of the incus.

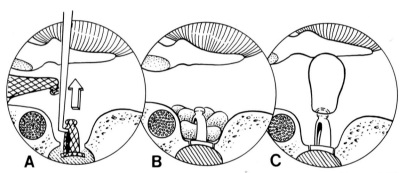

Figure 6-52

Figure 6-52A demonstrates the elevation of the stapes from its depressed position. Figure 6-52B demonstrates the placement of Gelfoam packing about the repositioned stapes. In cases where multiple disruptions have occurred, it is prudent to reestablish the position of the stapes in the oval window niche in the primary procedure with reconstruction of the ossicular chain in a subsequent operation. In Figure 6-52A the incus has been left within the confines of the epitympanic space for preservation and subsequent use. Figure 6-52C demonstrates the use of a sculptured incus autograft in the reconstruction of ossicular continuity.

Figure 6-53 demonstrates the placement of a fat-wire malleolar-to-oval window prosthesis in light of the disruption and absence of the stapes suprastructure and incus.

Fixation (see Chapter 9).

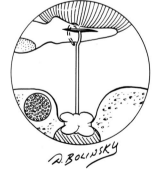

Figure 6-53

COMBINED OSSICULAR PROBLEMS

Fixation of Malleus, Incus, and Stapes

On occasion, multiple ossicular fixations are present. Disarticulation of fixed ossicles may traumatize the vestibule and subsequently the inner ear; therefore, it is often prudent to separate the incudostapedial joint prior to manipulation and mobilization of either the malleus or the incus (Figure 6-54).

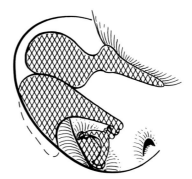

Figure 6-54

Note that the incudostapedial joint shown in Figure 6-55 is atraumatically separated. This will reduce the possibility of traumatizing the inner ear when manipulating the incus and malleus.

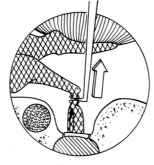

Figure 6-55

Figure 6-56A shows that the incus has been removed. The malleus head is carefully amputated. Care should be taken not to disrupt the tympanic membrane. This is of paramount importance. The stapes and footplate are then removed (Figure 6-56B).

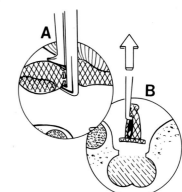

Figure 6-56

A malleus-to-oval window prosthesis wire is placed (Figure 6-57A). Autogenous tissue is placed within the oval-window niche. A TORP is placed (Figure 6-57B). Again, autogenous material (vein or fascia) may be insinuated in the oval window niche while cartilage rests between the lateral portion of the TORP and the tympanic membrane.

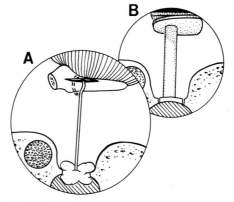

Figure 6-57

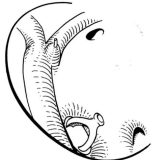

Figure 6-58

Absence of Malleus and Incus

Figure 6-58 demonstrates the absence of both malleus and incus.

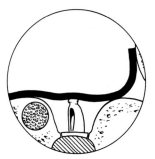

Figure 6-59

Figure 6-59 shows placement of autogenous graft material in a Type III tympanoplasty on the mobile stapes suprastructure.

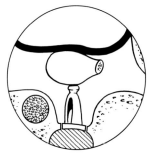

Figure 6-60

Figure 6-60 demonstrates the use of a homograft incus that has been sculptured to create a larger tympanic space.

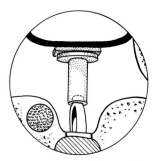

Figure 6-61

Figure 6-61 illustrates placement of a PORP; again, the objective is to create a larger tympanic space.

Absence of Malleus, Incus, and Suprastructure of Stapes (Mobile Footplate)

Figure 6-62 demonstrates absence of malleus, incus, and stapes suprastructure.

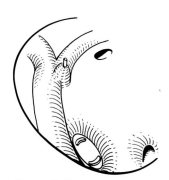

Figure 6-62

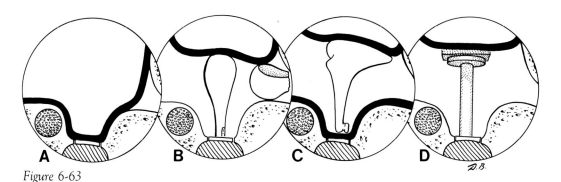

Figure 6-63

Figure 6-63 shows placement of a graft directly on the mobile footplate, as routinely performed with Type IV tympanoplasty. Figure 6-63B illustrates placement of a sculptured malleus columella strut between graft and mobile footplate, along with a head of the malleus, which creates an air space in the mesotympanum. Figure 6-63C shows placement of an incus columella homograft and Figure 6-63D, placement of a TORP. Note the positioning of cartilage between the tympanic membrane and lateral portion of the TORP.

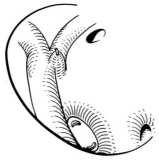

Figure 6-64

Absence of Malleus, Incus, and Suprastructure of Stapes (Fixed Footplate)

Figure 6-64 shows absence of malleus, incus, stapes suprastructure, and fixation of footplate.

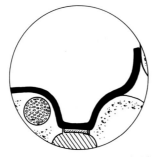

Figure 6-65

A Type IV tympanoplasty may be performed in the primary procedure as demonstrated in Figure 6-65.

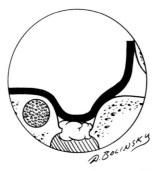

Figure 6-66

Stapedectomy and insertion of autogenous material are performed in a later operation (Type Vb) as shown in Figure 6-66.

An alternative to this technique would be the performance of a fenestration procedure (Type Va) shown in Table 4-1, Figure Va.

PROBLEMS AND SOLUTIONS

The otologist must be aware of the fact that technique and appropriate choice of grafting material play a large part in the success of graft placement. Attention to the finest details of size and location of graft placement will contribute to a successful outcome; conversely, failure to follow meticulous procedure principles will most assuredly result in a failed graft.

A lateralized incus homograft is demonstrated in Figure 6-67. Conversely, retraction may displace the medial end of the homograft into the vestibule. A connective tissue graft should be placed over the oval window.

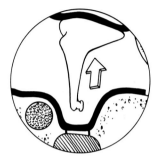

Figure 6-67

Figure 6-68 shows a sculptured malleus homograft that has lateralized.

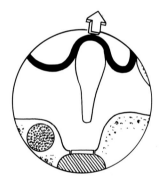

Figure 6-68

The malleus-to-oval window wire piston prosthesis placement is technically difficult. The shaft and crook shown in Figure 6-69 are lateralized. Commonly, the wire has not been crimped well to the manubrium (see section on stapedectomy in fenestrated ear in Chapter 9).

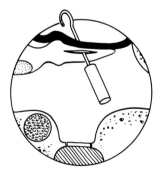

Figure 6-69

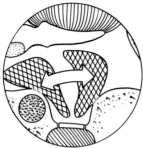

Figure 6-70

A sculptured incus homograft or autograft may become fixed to the facial ridge, cochleariform process, the promontory, or the bony rim of the annulus (Figure 6-70). Retraction may separate the interposition graft incus from the malleus laterally.

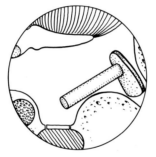
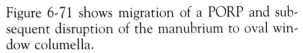

Figure 6-71

Figure 6-71 shows migration of a PORP and subsequent disruption of the manubrium to oval window columella.

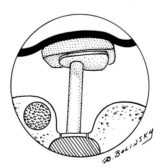

Figure 6-72

As shown in Figure 6-72, the problem illustrated in Figure 6-71 may be overcome by placing a piece of cartilage between the head of the PORP and the tympanic membrane.

REFERENCES

1. Austin, D. F.: Ossicular Reconstruction. *Arch. Otolaryngol.*, 94:525–535, 1971.
2. Brackmann, D. E. and Sheehy, J. L.: Tympanoplasty: TORPs and PORPs. *Laryngoscope*, 89:108–114, 1979.
3. Cody, R. T. and Taylor, W. F.: Tympanoplasty: Long-Term Hearing Results with Incus Grafts. *Laryngoscope*, 83:852–864, 1973.
4. English, G. E., Hildyard, V. H., Hemenway, W. G., *et al.*: Autograft and Homograft Incus Transpositions in Chronic Otitis Media. *Laryngoscope*, 81:1434–1445, 1971.
5. Hough, J. V. D.: Incudostapedial Joint Separation. *Laryngoscope*, 69:644–664, 1959.
6. Lesinski, S. G. (Ed.): Symposium on Homograft Tympanoplasty. *Otolaryngol. Clin. N. Am.* 10(3), October 1977.
7. Pennington, C. L.: Incus Interposition Techniques. *Ann. Otol. Rhinol. Laryngol.*, 82:518–531, 1973.
8. Shea, J.: Plastipore Total Ossicular Replacement Prosthesis. *Laryngoscope*, 86:239–240, 1976.
9. Shea, J. and Emmett, J. R.: Biocompatible Ossicular Implants. *Arch. Otolaryngol.*, 104:191–196, 1978.
10. Smyth, G. D. L.: Five-Year Report on Partial Ossicular Replacement Prosthesis and Total Ossicular Replacement Prostheses. *Otolaryngol. Head Neck Surg.*, 90:343–346, 1982.

7

Homograft Tympanoplasty

Eiji Yanagisawa
Myles L. Pensak

The introduction of homograft tympanoplasty by Chalat in 1964[2] represents a small but significant chapter in the annals of transplantation and otologic reconstructive surgery. Fundamental to an appreciation of the homograft tympanoplasty is an understanding of the principles of transplantation immunobiology and "traditional" tympanoplastic surgical indications, goals, and techniques. A description of these thoughts is beyond the scope of this chapter; however, we encourage the reader to pursue the classic articles and texts on these topics.

Table 7-1 defines several terms that are used frequently when discussing grafts and the source from which they are derived. Materials to be used for homograft transplantation may originate from either preserved material obtained in the operating room or the cadaver.

Table 7-1
Definitions

Autograft: Describes a Graft Taken from One Site of an Individual and Placed on Another Site of the Same Individual

Isograft: Describes a Graft Exchanged Between Genetically Identical Individuals

Allograft (Homograft): Describes a Graft Transfer from One Individual to Another (Species-Specific)

Xenograft: Describes a Graft Between Different Species

Orthotopic Graft: Describes a Graft Transplanted to Its Normal Anatomic Environment

Heterotopic Graft: Describes a Graft Transplanted into a Nonanatomic Environment for the Grafted Material

The search for a satisfactory preservative for homo-graft material hampered progress. The introduction of buffered formaldehyde solution by Perkins in 1970[11] improved the success rate of homograft tympanoplasty.

Four clinically effective preservatives are (1) 70% alcohol solution;[17] (2) 4% buffered formaldehyde fixation, 0.5% buffered formaldehyde preservation;[6,12,13] (3) 4% buffered formaldehyde fixation, 1:5000 Cialit (Solium 2-ethylmercurithiobenzoxazole-5 carboxylate) preservation;[7] and (4) Cialit fixation and preservation.[1]

Furthermore, various physical techniques have been described for preservation, such as freezing by refrigeration, deep freezing, heating, irradiation, and drying.

Indications for homograft tympanoplasty include previous failure with standard tympanoplasty, such as recurrent perforations, graft lateralization, and canal stenosis (see Chapters 5 and 6); high risk of failure with standard tympanoplasty, including total or subtotal tympanic membrane perforation with absent malleus and/or anterior annulus; and reconstruction of the radical mastoidectomy cavity or of congenital aural atresia.

The use of homograft material for middle-ear reconstruction affords the otologic surgeon one more means of restoring a functional middle ear to those patients who have had significant disruption of their air-conducting mechanisms. Although we currently have the means for performing homograft tympanoplasty, there are several economic and ethical factors involved in the use of homograft material. Fortunately, thanks to the work of Smith, Lesinski, Perkins, and others who are active in the functions of the Regional Ear Banks, both patients and surgeons can, under the proper circumstances, make use of homograft material for tympanoplasty.

ACQUISITION OF TRANSPLANT MATERIAL

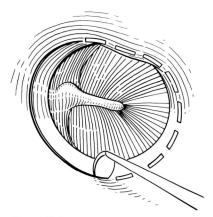

Figure 7-1

FROM CADAVER

Transmeatal Approach

A circumferential incision is made 0.5 cm from the annulus tympanicus (Figure 7-1).

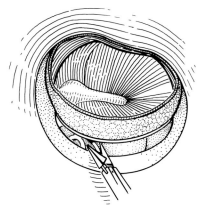

A tympanomeatal flap is elevated in both the pars tensa and pars flaccida regions, including the fibrous annulus (Figure 7-2). The chorda tympani nerve is severed.

Figure 7-2

Attendent malleolar ligaments (posterior and anterior) along with the tensor tympani are divided (Figure 7-3). The tympanic membrane with or without the malleus is delivered. After fixation (4% buffered formaldehyde) and preservation (0.5% buffered formaldehyde), the squamous epithelium of the tympanic membrane is removed before homograft use.

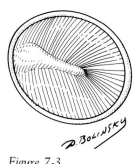

Figure 7-3

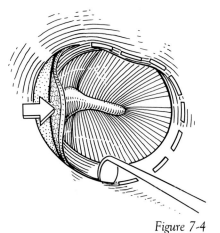

Figure 7-4

TRANSCRANIAL APPROACH (MARQUET AND GLASSCOCK)

A circumferential incision is made 0.5 cm from the annulus tympanicus. The fibrous annulus is carefully preserved with the elevator (Figure 7-4).

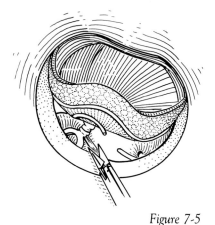

Figure 7-5

The chorda tympani nerve is sectioned (Figure 7-5), and the stapedius tendon is divided without disruption of the incudostapedial joint.

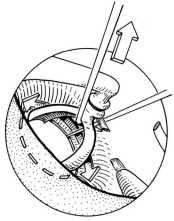

Figure 7-6

Using a sharp needle or sickle knife, the annular ligament of the footplate is freed with gentle posterior to anterior sweeping motions about the stapes footplate (Figure 7-6). A 1-mm right-angle hook carefully elevates the stapes from the oval window niche. It should be remembered that the ossicular chain is still fixed in the epitympanum; and therefore, no attempt should be made to remove the stapes.

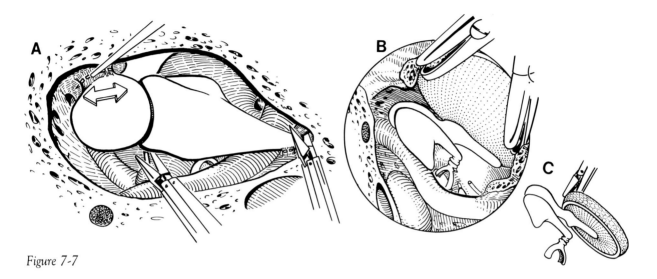

Figure 7-7

The epitympanum is now exposed with burrs and curettes (Figure 7-7A). The malleolar ligaments are severed. The tensor tympani tendon is also divided.

Medium-sized bone biting forceps or a drill are used to remove any excess bone that may inhibit removal of the tympano-ossicular complex (Figure 7-7B). The tympanic membrane and ossicles are removed, fixed, and preserved (Figure 7-7C). The squamous epithelium of the tympanic membrane and the canal skin are removed prior to use.

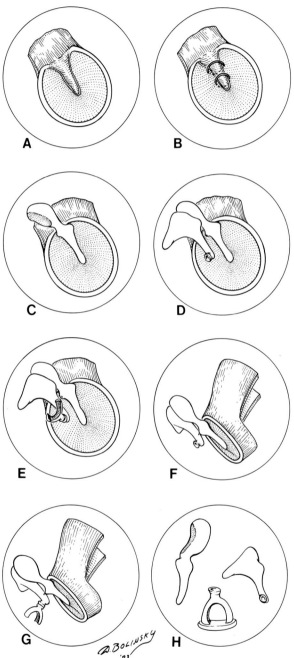

FROM TEMPORAL BONE BANK

Homograft material can now be obtained from the existing otologic tissue banks such as the Cincinnati Ear Bank, Cincinnati, Ohio; The Ear Bank of Project Hear, Palo Alto, California; and Northern California Transplant Bank, San Jose, California.

The following homograft materials are available through the Ear Bank of Project Hear: tympanic membrane (Figure 7-8A), tympanic membrane with suture slings (B), tympanic membrane with malleus (C), tympanic membrane with malleus-incus (en bloc) (D), tympanic membrane with malleus-incus and crural segment (E), tympanic membrane with malleus-incus (en bloc) with long canal cuff (F), tympanic membrane with malleus-incus and crural segment with long canal cuff (G), and homograft ossicles (H).

Figure 7-8

SURGICAL TECHNIQUES

TYMPANIC HOMOGRAFT TYMPANOPLASTY

Marquet Technique

By use of a sickle knife, the squamous epithelium layer of the drum remnant is freshened and removed carefully preserving the fibrous drum layer (Figure 7-9).

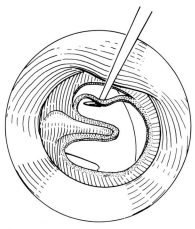

Figure 7-9

Incisions are made at 11, 2, and 7 o'clock positions from the bony sulcus, including the annulus (unless annular continuity is complete and the homograft is to be placed with an intact annulus), and carried from medial to lateral positions (Figure 7-10). (Modified from Marquet's original technique.)

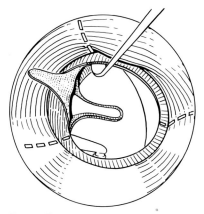

Figure 7-10

The squamous epithelium is elevated from the tympanic membrane and the anterior canal wall with annulus remnant separation (artist's view, Figure 7-11).

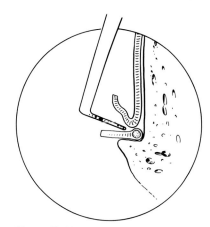

Figure 7-11

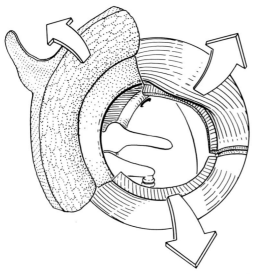

The flaps are reflected exposing the middle-ear space (Figure 7-12). Tympanosclerosis (if present) and annular remnants are removed.

Figure 7-12

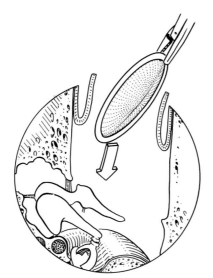

After the condition of the ossicles is established, the homograft tympanic membrane is introduced and placed in position, first on the manubrium and then on the short process of the malleus (Figure 7-13).

Figure 7-13

The annulus is placed in the bony sulcus from anterior to posterior (Figure 7-14).

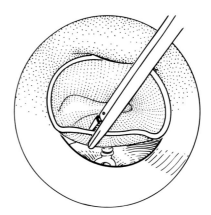

Figure 7-14

The canal flaps are returned to their anatomic positions (Figure 7-15).

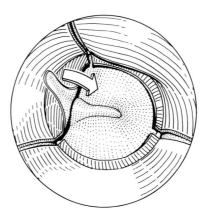

Figure 7-15

Figure 7-16 shows a cross section of the canal wall flaps overlapping the homograft tympanic membrane.

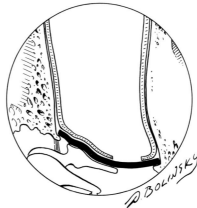

Figure 7-16

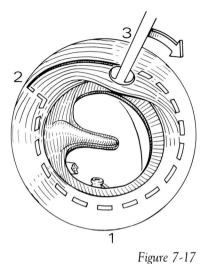

Figure 7-17

Wehrs Technique

Three canal wall incisions are made; the first along the tympanomastoid suture line, the second along the tympanosquamous suture line, and a third that joins these two (Figure 7-17).

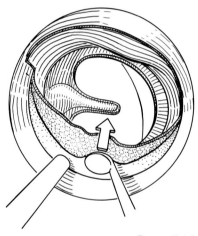

Figure 7-18

Canal skin is then elevated down to and including the squamous epithelium of the tympanic membrane remnant and removed (Figure 7-18).

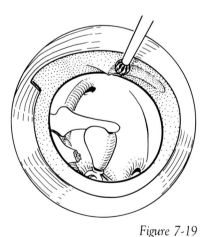

Figure 7-19

Optimal exposure is obtained by burring or curetting down all bony overhangs to visualize the anterior tympanic sulcus (Figure 7-19). Ossicular reconstruction is performed as indicated.

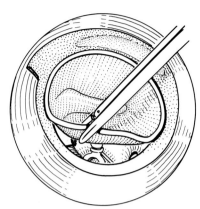

Figure 7-20

The homograft is placed over the remnant of the denuded tympanic membrane (Figure 7-20). All squamous epithelium material must be removed prior to grafting to avoid cholesteatoma formation.

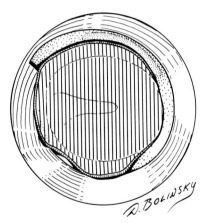

Figure 7-21

The canal skin is freshened and placed over the homograft (Figure 7-21). The skin may extend to the anterior canal wall, but should not blunt the acute anterior angle.

OSSICULAR HOMOGRAFT TYMPANOPLASTY

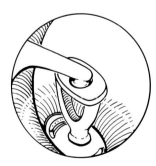

Figure 7-22

Variable success rates have been reported to obtain good hearing results with these techniques. The success generally reflects the skills and ingenuity of the surgeon and the middle-ear-space conditions.

Homograft stapes [(inverted) in Figure 7-22 (Marquet)] is positioned between the lenticular process of the incus and footplate of the stapes. Exact size measurement must be established prior to placement.

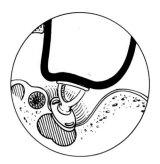

Figure 7-23 shows a modified Type IV tympano-plasty reconstruction employing the inverted stapes homograft.

Figure 7-23

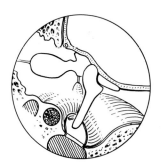

The sculptured malleus homograft is a dependable and versatile graft (Figure 7-24).

Figure 7-24

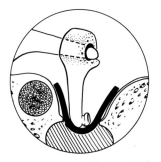

The sculptured incus with notch rests between the patient's oval window niche (with autogenous material placed) and the patient's incus [Figure 7-25 (Marquet)].

Figure 7-25

TYMPANIC-OSSICULAR HOMOGRAFT TYMPANOPLASTY (AFTER GLASSCOCK)

The external auditory canal is prepared (Figure 7-26). Incisions are made in the tympanosquamous and tympanomastoid suture lines. The vascular strip is retracted and preserved while the anterior canal wall skin is elevated, removed, and preserved to afford optimal exposure of the middle-ear space.

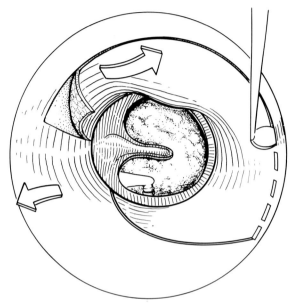

Figure 7-26

A postauricular incision is made, and the auricle is displaced anteriorly and the middle ear visualized (Figure 7-27).

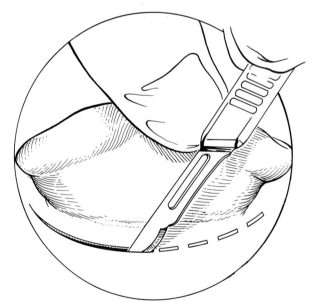

Figure 7-27

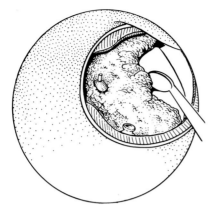

The tympanic cavity is inspected and diseased tissue is removed cautiously (Figure 7-28). Identification of the stapes remnant is sometimes difficult; however, the surgeon must exert minimal trauma to the footplate to ensure a subsequent optimal functional result.

Figure 7-28

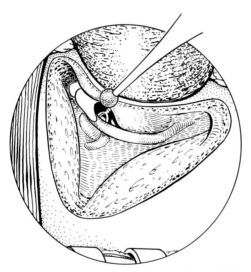

A cortical mastoidectomy is performed with cutting burrs (Figure 7-29). The facial recess is opened with a diamond burr.

Figure 7-29

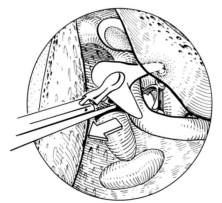

The incus is removed (Figure 7-30). Usually the lenticular process has been eroded by the chronic inflammatory process; however, in cases where it remains attached to the capitulum of the stapes, separation should be atraumatic.

Figure 7-30

The malleus is removed (Figure 7-31).

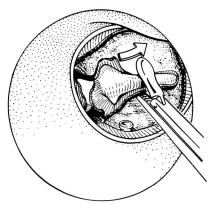

Figure 7-31

The stapes (or remnant) is palpated and a mobile footplate appreciated. Silastic sheeting is introduced through the facial recess (Figure 7-32). The Silastic will serve as a foundation for promoting homograft stability.

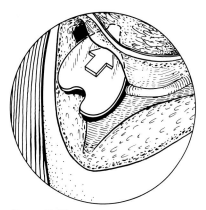

Figure 7-32

Gelfoam moistened with antibiotic solution is introduced over the Silastic sheeting (Figure 7-33). A notch made in the Silastic sheeting and not covered by Gelfoam allows for mobility of the stapes capitulum and the lenticular process of the incus.

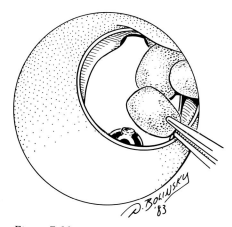

Figure 7-33

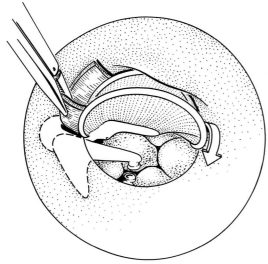

Figure 7-34

The homograft is placed (Figure 7-34).

Ossicular continuity is demonstrated in Figure 7-35A. Gelfoam is placed about the incus for support and to obviate the problem of incudostapedial disarticulation. The canal skin is returned to its anatomic position while the vascular strip is reflected into place (Figure 7-35B). A free piece of canal skin overlies the pars flaccida. Canal skin may overlie but not completely cover the homograft tympanic membrane.

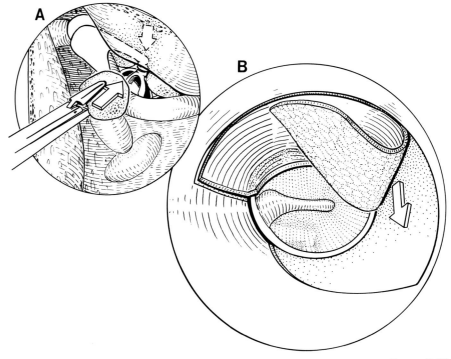

Figure 7-35

Gelfoam packing is applied lateral to the graft (Figure 7-36).

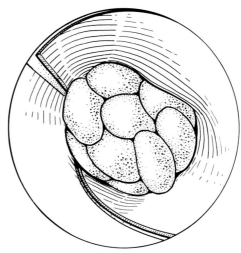

Figure 7-36

A rosebud-style double-packing technique employing Owens silk and Vaseline gauze impregnated with antibiotic solution is placed in the canal (Figure 7-37). A mastoid-style dressing is applied following the closure of the postauricular incision.

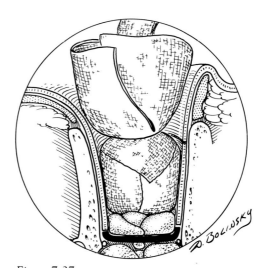

Figure 7-37

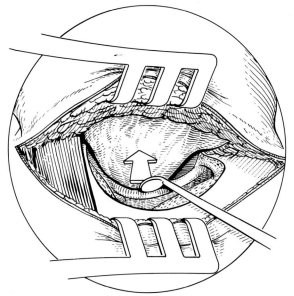

Figure 7-38

HOMOGRAFT RECONSTRUCTION OF RADICAL MASTOIDECTOMY CAVITY (AFTER MARQUET)

A standard postauricular incision is made approximately 1.5 cm behind the auricle (Figure 7-38). Self-retaining retractors are placed and soft tissues elevated from the mastoid, antrum, attic, and mesotympanum, including the drum in an anterior direction. The surgeon should clearly establish that no inflammation or infected tissue remains sequestered in the oval window, round window, or sinus tympani regions. In the mastoid cavity proper, new bone should be removed only if it permits access to sequestered pathology.

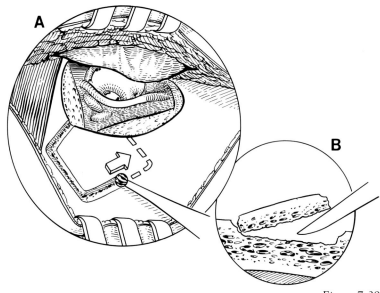

Figure 7-39

With the mastoid cavity and tympanum evacuated of diseased tissue, a cortical bone graft is harvested (Figure 7-39A). An outline of the graft is made with a fine cutting burr posterior and superior to the recesses of the defined mastoid cavity. Once defined, the cortical bone graft is removed with a chisel (Figure 7-39B).

The bone graft is burred to conform and contour the posterior canal wall that it will form (Figure 7-40).

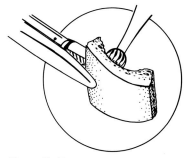

Figure 7-40

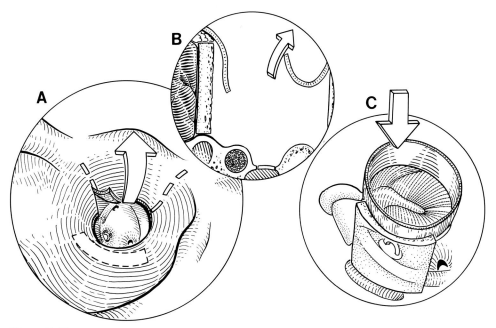

Figure 7-41

Incisions are made at the 12 o'clock and 4 o'clock positions from the bony annulus laterally along the anterior canal wall (Figure 7-41A). A flap is elevated and reflected laterally. With anterior and posterior canal skin flaps elevated, the mastoid is obliterated by musculoplasty, and the contoured cortical bone is placed posterior to the facial ridge (Figure 7-41B) The chosen homograft (drum and ossicles) are placed with the external canal skin sleeve carefully lying on the posterior bony canal wall autograft (Figure 7-41C).

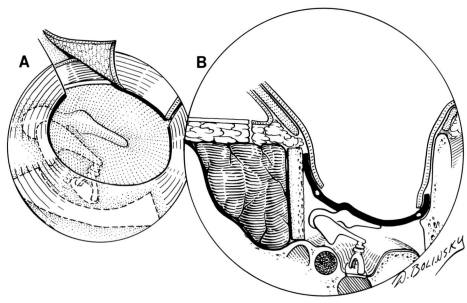

Figure 7-42

The skin flaps are reflected back into their anatomic positions overlying the canal sleeves of the homograft (Figure 7-42A). Figure 7-42B shows cross sections of the musculoplastic obliteration of the mastoid cavity. The bony autograft reconstructing the posterior canal wall and the skin flaps overlying the posterior and anterior aspects of the homograft tympanic membrane are seen. Several authors have recommended covering the homograft with fascia,[3] which is then covered by the anterior and posterior canal skin flaps.

DISCUSSION

Refinement and alteration in techniques for any given procedure reflects the successes and failures of the current practice. Homograft tympanoplastic techniques (especially major procedures involving the drum and ossicles) are not as yet widely employed. Several reasons for this appear to be success of autogenous grafting materials and prosthetic materials, inexperience and lack of familiarity with homografts on the part of the general otolaryngologist, and variable reported success with homograft materials by those who have used them extensively.

Problems with homografts may be defined as occurring to the drum or drum ossicle complex or ossicles. One salient figure reported by Marquet was that 52 percent in a series of 140 patients had recurrent disease that was not related to the homograft but was ascribed to infection, cholesteatoma, eustachian tube dysfunction, or tympanosclerosis. This posits the most important fact—specifically, that if the tympanic cavity, by virtue of its final preoperative status, is not void of disease or is not physiologically amenable to grafting, no reconstruction, homograft, or autograft will ensure success. Finally, both surgeon and patient must be cognizant of the fact that homografts cannot offer a panacea for the patient with chronic ear disease.

REFERENCES

1. Brandow, E. C.: Homograft Tympanic Membrane Transplant in Myringoplasty. *Trans. Am. Acad. Ophthal. Otolaryngol.* 73:825–835, 1969.
2. Chalat, N. L.: Tympanic Membrane Transplant. *Harper Hosp. Bull.,* 22:27–34, 1964.
3. Glasscock, M. E. and House, W. F.: Homograft Reconstruction of the Middle Ear. *Laryngoscope,* 78:1219, 1968.
4. Glasscock, M. E., III, House, W. F., Graham, M.: Homograft Transplants to the Middle Ear. A Follow-up Report. *Laryngoscope,* 82:868–881, 1972.
5. Lesinski, S. G. (Ed.): Symposium on Homograft Tympanoplasty. *Otolaryngol. Clin. N. Am.,* 10(3), October 1977.
6. Lesinski, S. G.: Indications for Homograft Tympanoplasty—A Clinical Study. *Otolaryngol. Clin. N. Am.,* 10(3):507–515, 1977.
7. Marquet, J.: Reconstructive Micro-surgery of the Eardrum by Means of a Tympanic Membrane Homograft: Preliminary Report. *Acta Otolaryngol.,* 62:459–464, 1966.
8. Marquet, J. F. E.: Homografts in Tympanoplasty and Other Middle Ear Surgery. In: Operative Surgery, J. Ballantyne (Ed.). Butterworths, London, 100–115, 1976.
9. Marquet, J.: Twelve Years' Experience with Homograft Tympanoplasty. *Otolaryngol. Clin. N. Am.,* 10(3):581, 1977.
10. Perkins, R.: Human Homograft Otologic Tissue Transplantation: Buffered Formaldehyde Preparation. *Trans. Am. Acad. Ophthal. Otolaryngol.* 74:278–282, 1970.
11. Perkins, R.: The Ear Bank of Project HEAR. *Trans. Am. Acad. Ophthal. Otolaryngol.,* 80:23–29, 1975.
12. Perkins, R.: Otologic Homograft Indications, Techniques and Anatomical and Functional Results. *Trans. Am. Acad. Ophthal. Otolaryngol.,* 80:44–46, 1975.
13. Pulec, J. L.: Homograft Tympanoplasty Techniques and Results for Restoration of Hearing. *Otolaryngol. Clin. N. Am.,* 10:553–540, 1977.
14. Smith, M. F. W.: An Otologic Tissue Bank. *Trans. Am. Acad. Ophthal. Otolaryngol.,* 76:134–141, 1972.
15. Smith, M. F. W. and Downey, D.: Otologic Homograft Indications, Techniques and Anatomic and Functional Results. *Trans. Am. Acad. Ophthal. Otolaryngol.,* 80:47–51, 1975.
16. Wehrs, R. E.: Homograft Tympanic Membrane in Tympanoplasty. *Arch. Otolaryngol.* 93:132–139, 1971.
17. Wehrs, R. E.: The Homograft Notched Incus in Tympanoplasty. *Arch. Otolaryngol.,* 100:251–255, 1974.
18. Wehrs, R. E.: Surgical Techniques of Homograft Tympanoplasty. *Otolaryngol. Clin. N. Am.,* 10:517–526, 1977.

8

Surgery for Middle-Ear
——————Congenital Cholesteatoma——————

"Congenital cholesteatoma auris," an alternate term for middle-ear congenital cholesteatoma, implies a cholesteatoma that develops behind an intact tympanic membrane in a patient without previous history of aural infections, and presumably arises from embryonal inclusion of squamous epithelium or undifferentiated tissue that changes to squamous epithelium in the developing temporal bone.[4]

TRANSCANAL APPROACH

A small-sized congenital cholesteatoma of the middle ear can be removed through the transcanal approach. A whitish mass can often be seen through an intact tympanic membrane.

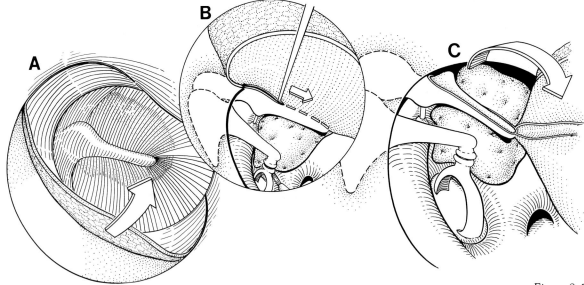

Figure 8-1

Figure 8-1A shows a tympanotomy incision similar to that for a stapedectomy is made starting from the 6 o'clock to the 12 o'clock positions, on to the 2 o'clock position. The flap should be wide in the attic area. The tympanomeatal flap is elevated and the middle ear exposed. The flap is separated from the short process and the upper surface of the manubrium of the malleus. The insert to Figure 8-1B shows a method of separation of the tympanic membrane from the manubrium of the malleus. The periosteal incision is made along the upper border of the manubrium near the tympanic membrane, and the membrane is carefully separated from the manubrium by using a sickle knife. The flap is elevated downward and placed over the inferior half of the tympanic membrane (Figure 8-1C). Note that the tympanic membrane is still attached to the umbo. This will prevent postoperative lateral displacement of the tympanic membrane and will maintain its conical shape. The cholesteatoma is limited to the anterior superior quadrant of the tympanic cavity and is well exposed. The chorda tympani nerve is identified and stretched somewhat and placed in the superior portion of the ear canal (not shown in Figure 8-1). If its presence compromises excision of the cholesteatoma, it should be sectioned and excised.

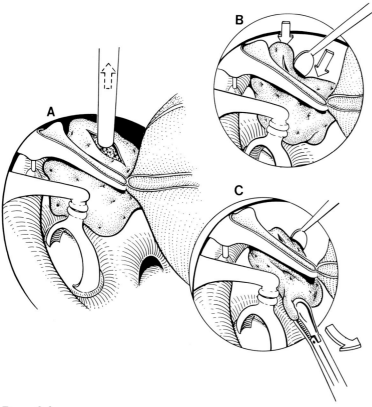

Figure 8-2

Through a small incision, the middle-ear cholesteatoma is decompressed (Figure 8-2A). A No. 7
suction tube is inserted into the cholesteatomatous
mass, and the contents are suctioned away. The
decompressed sac is then elevated from the middle-
ear mucosa from anteriorly to posteriorly (Figure
2B). With extreme care taken not to injure the
mobile stapes, the mass is grasped with cup forceps
and removed (Figure 8-2C). It is important at this
time to inspect the medial aspect of the middle ear
to see whether there are any remnants of the cho-
lesteatomous sac; if so, they are completely excised.

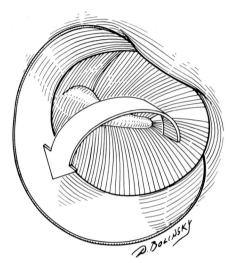

Figure 8-3

The tympanic membrane is then brought back to its anatomic position, and the ear canal is packed with Gelfoam and antibiotic impregnated ½-inch-wide Vaseline gauze (Figure 8-3).

ALTERNATIVE PROCEDURES

ENDAURAL ATTICOTYMPANOTOMY (DERLACKI)

Derlacki[4] applies this technique for congenital cholesteatoma of the middle ear that extends into the attic. The author prefers to use a combined transcanal postauricular approach.

COMBINED TRANSCANAL AND POSTAURICULAR ATTICOTYMPANOTOMY

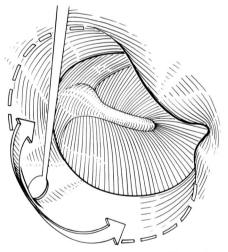

Figure 8-4

An exploratory tympanotomy is performed through a transcanal approach first (Figure 8-4). A long tympanomeatal flap is made starting approximately 3 mm away from the annulus tympanicus, extending down to the 6 o'clock position and upward through the 12 o'clock to the 1 o'clock positions. The flap should be large enough to cover an atticotomy defect that will be created to remove the incus and head of the malleus if necessary, as well as to remove the extension of the middle-ear cholesteatoma from the attic.

The tympanomeatal flap is elevated and the middle ear exposed. The size and extent of the cholesteatoma is ascertained. When it is found to extend into the attic, and when it is impossible to remove the cholesteatoma through the transcanal approach, a combination of transcanal and postauricular approaches is carried out (Figure 8-5).

Through a standard postauricular incision, the posterior membranous canal wall is incised at the level of the cortex of the mastoid (Figure 8-6). The incision is extended from 12 o'clock to the 6 o'clock position. Care must be exercised not to cut anteriorly into the anterior canal wall skin when the canal is entered.

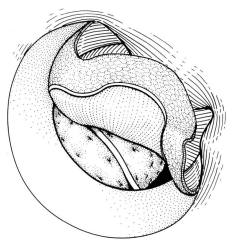

Figure 8-5

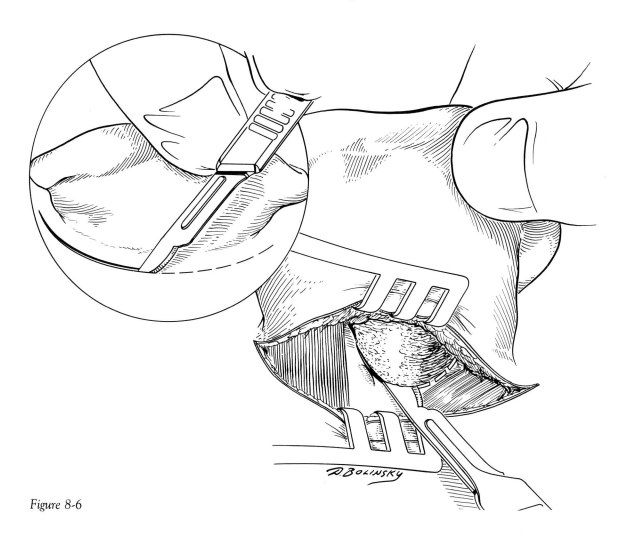

Figure 8-6

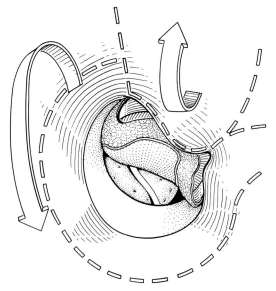

Two vertical (medial to lateral) incisions are then made at the 2 o'clock and 6 o'clock positions (Figure 8-7). These incisions are connected medially.

Figure 8-7

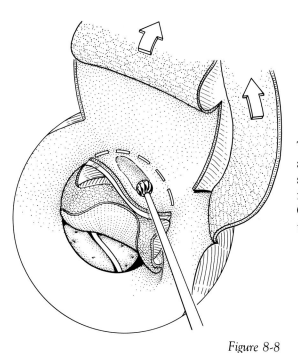

The anterior canal wall skin is elevated laterally and reflected (Figure 8-8). The posterior canal wall skin (including superior skin) is elevated and reflected as a laterally and inferiorly based pedicle. Often a bony overhang is appreciated on the anterior canal wall.

Figure 8-8

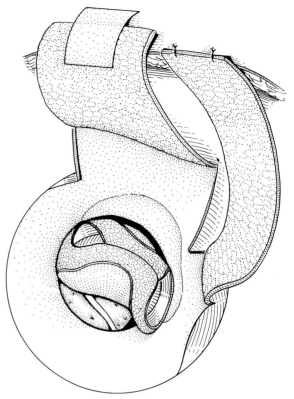

The anterior canal skin flap is retracted carefully out of the field while the laterally and inferiorly based pedicle is sutured to the anterior skin flap to prevent avulsion with 4-0 catgut sutures (Figure 8-9). The anterior bony overhang may be burred down to permit optimal visualization of the tympanum.

Figure 8-9

Figure 8-10 illustrates an artist's concept of the canal and bony overhang (dotted line) and the relative position of the cholesteatoma. The size of the cholesteatoma dictates the feasibility of a transcanal excision of the cholesteatoma or the need for a combined approach.

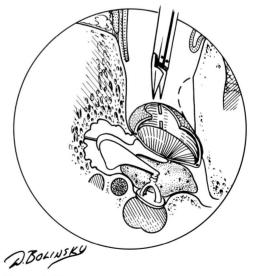

Figure 8-10

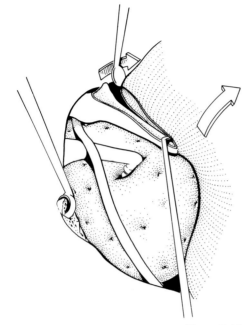

Figure 8-11

Often the posterior bony canal must be taken down either by curet or burr (Figure 8-11). As the position of the stapes suprastructure may be obscured by the cholesteatoma, extreme caution must be exercised. The tympanic membrane is scored by a sickle knife and the drum gently elevated off the manubrium of the malleus. The tympanic membrane flap is turned anteriorly and inferiorly.

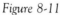

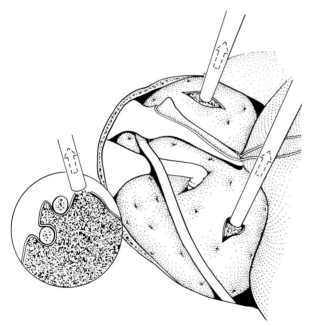

Figure 8-12

Atticotomy is performed for exposure as required. The cholesteatoma is decompressed by incision and suction evacuation.

Figure 8-12 shows the cholesteatoma as it often inserts itself between the malleus and incus (insert).

The cholesteatoma sac is carefully elevated in a posterior-to-anterior direction (Figure 8-13). The incudostapedial joint is disarticulated to avoid trauma to the footplate and inner ear. The insert depicts the cholesteatoma mass as it juxtaposes the stapes footplate and oval window extending medially to the promontory.

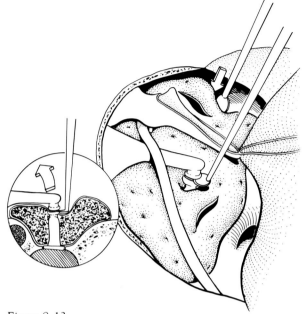

Figure 8-13

The cholesteatoma is mobilized toward the stapes and excised around the stapes (Figure 8-14A). The remaining cholesteatoma around the stapes is carefully removed (Figure 8-14B). Fine dissection may be accomplished by using an incudostapedial joint knife and a No. 20 suction tube under a 16× magnification.

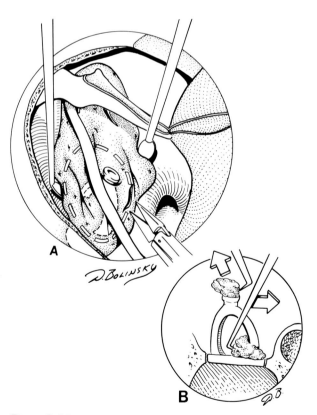

Figure 8-14

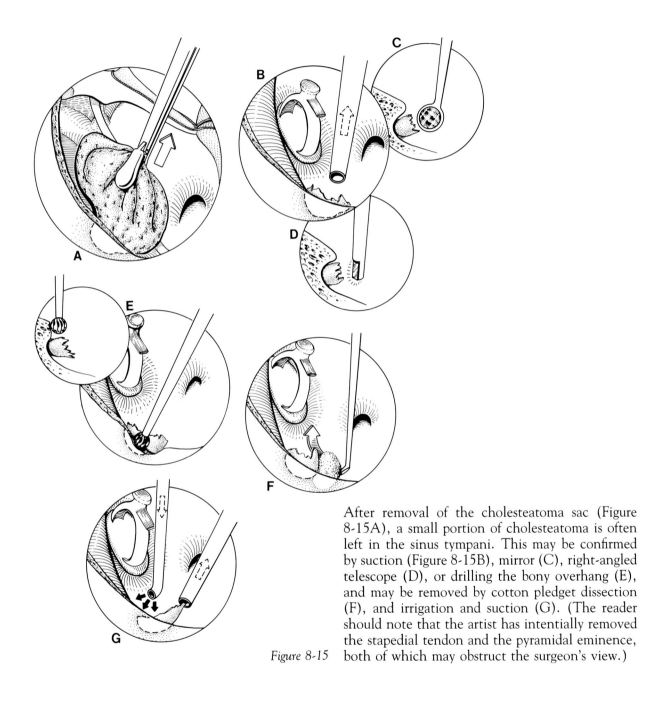

After removal of the cholesteatoma sac (Figure 8-15A), a small portion of cholesteatoma is often left in the sinus tympani. This may be confirmed by suction (Figure 8-15B), mirror (C), right-angled telescope (D), or drilling the bony overhang (E), and may be removed by cotton pledget dissection (F), and irrigation and suction (G). (The reader should note that the artist has intentially removed the stapedial tendon and the pyramidal eminence, both of which may obstruct the surgeon's view.)

Figure 8-15

After the cholesteatoma is completely evacuated and the footplate found mobile, a sculptured incus may be placed between the stapes and malleus to establish ossicular continuity (Figure 8-16). Gelfoam is then placed in the middle ear.

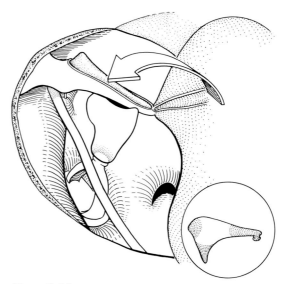

Figure 8-16

The tympanotomy flap is then returned to its anatomic position (Figure 8-17). A temporalis fascia graft is placed over the atticotomy defect and medial to the tympanic membrane.

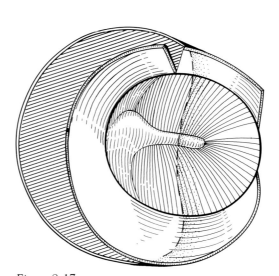

Figure 8-17

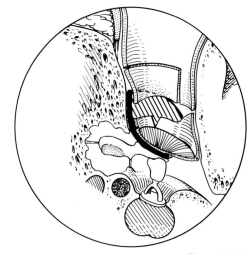

Figure 8-18 represents an artist's view of the completed combined approach. This figure should be compared with Figure 8-10.

Figure 8-18

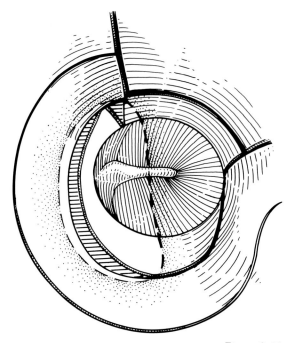

The meatal flaps are brought back to their original positions (Figure 8-19). Note that the temporalis fascia graft (dotted line in Figure 8-19) is placed medially to the tympanic membrane.

Figure 8-19

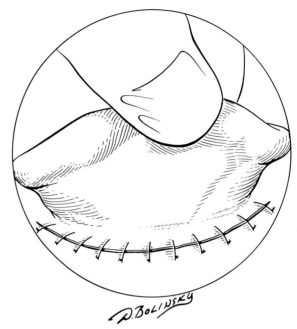

The postauricular incision is closed (Figure 8-20). The canal is packed with antibiotic impregnated Gelfoam and double packings and a mastoid dressing is applied.

Figure 8-20

REFERENCES

1. Cawthorne, T. and Griffith, A.: Primary Cholesteatoma of the Temporal Bone. *Arch. Otolaryngol.*, 73:252–261, 1961.
2. Derlacki, E. L. and Clemis, J. D.: Congenital Cholesteatoma of the Middle Ear and Mastoid. *Ann Otol. Rhinol. Laryngol.*, 74:706–727, 1965.
3. Derlacki, E. L., Harrison, W. H., and Clemis, J. D.: Congenital Cholesteatoma of the Middle Ear and Mastoid: A Second Report Presenting Seven Additional Cases. *Laryngoscope*, 78:1050–1078, 1968.
4. Derlacki, E. L.: Congenital Cholesteatoma of the Middle Ear and Mastoid, A Third Report. *Arch. Otolaryngol.*, 97:177–182, 1973.
5. House, J. W. and Sheehy, J. L.: Cholesteatoma with Intact Tympanic Membrane: A Report of 41 Cases. *Laryngoscope*, 90:70–75, 1980.
6. Shambaugh, G. E., Jr. and Glasscock, M. E., III: Surgery of the Ear, 3rd ed. Saunders, Philadelphia, 1980.

9
━━━━━━━━━━━Stapedectomy━━━━━━━━━━━

In 1878 Kessel performed the first stapes mobilization, and in 1890 Miot reported 200 stapes mobilizations. In 1892 Blake of Boston removed a stapes to improve hearing, and in 1893 Jack reported a series of cases of extraction of the stapes. Ever since the revival of stapes mobilization by Rosen in 1952[17] and stapedectomy by Shea in 1958,[20] many different techniques of stapes surgery for otosclerosis have been designed. These techniques include stapedectomy with fat-wire prosthesis,[18] stapedectomy with preformed wire-Gelfoam prosthesis,[10] stapedectomy with piston,[18,20] interposition technique,[15] partial stapedectomy,[9] posterior arch stapedectomy,[8] footplate fragmentation technique,[11] small fenestra stapedectomy (stapedotomy), and laser stapedectomy.[14]

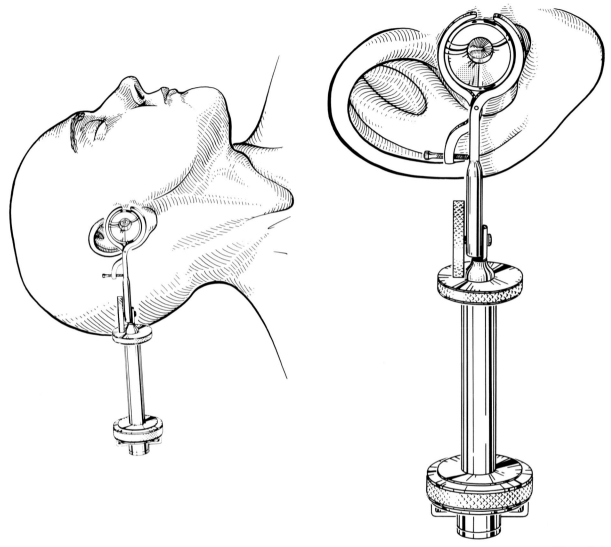

Figure 9-1

SURGICAL TECHNIQUES

TOTAL STAPEDECTOMY (SCHUKNECHT)

The ear is prepared with an antiseptic solution and draped. The external auditory canal is carefully cleaned. The patient's head is positioned in such a way that the posterior half of the tympanic membrane and the medial portion of the posterior canal wall are well visualized through the surgical microscope (Figure 9-1). The use of an ear speculum holder at this point is recommended for surgeons with limited experience to permit bimanual manipulation of the dissecting instruments and suction; more experienced surgeons prefer to use the speculum holder later in the procedure.

The procedure can be done under either local or
general anesthesia (Figure 9-2). In either case, the
ear canal is injected with 1% lidocaine (Xylocaine)
with epinephrine 1:100,000 dilution at the point
indicated in the cartilaginous canal with a 27-gauge
needle. The ear lobe is also injected at this time.

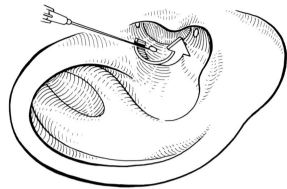

Figure 9-2

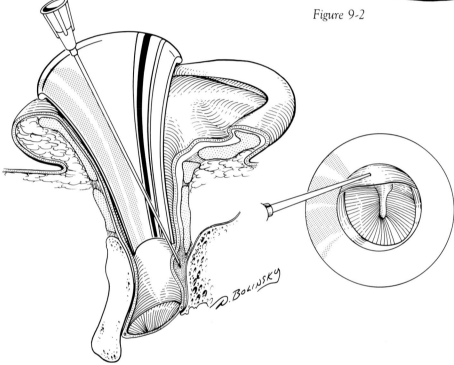

Figure 9-3

Additional injection is made in the vascular strip
with a 30-gauge needle until the blanching of the
canal skin down to the annulus is observed (Figure
9-3 insert). The injection should be done in an
atraumatic manner. The needle bevel must be flush
against the canal wall, parallel to the long axis of
the canal. Failure to do this will result in tearing
of the thin canal wall skin or precipitate bleeding
and bleb formation.

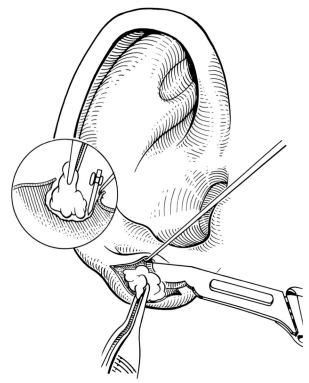

For the surgeon who employs a fat-wire prosthesis, the graft material is best obtained while the local anesthetic is taking effect (Figure 9-4). The incision is closed with 5-0 nylon sutures.

Figure 9-4

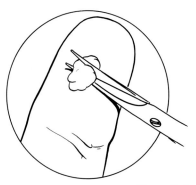

Placement of the fat on a slightly moistened index finger will ensure its safe transport to the "back table" (Figure 9-5). The surgeon's gloves should be washed with a damp cloth prior to handling of the fat to avoid introducing any foreign body contamination (talc) into the fat. Today many surgeons employ commercially manufactured stapes prostheses.

Figure 9-5

After trimming any traumatized fat, the tissue is placed over the edge of the stapes prosthesis die, and a loop of stainless steel wire [0.004 inch, 38 g or 0.005 inch, 36 g] is placed about the fat (2 mm × 3 mm) and secured. The author prefers the 0.005 with wire (Figure 9-6).

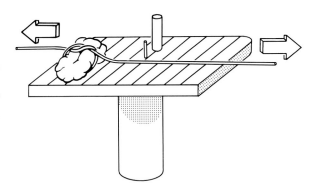

Figure 9-6

With the short post closest to the surgeon, the wire to the right of the fatty tissue is turned about the longer post 360° and held tight as it is placed flat on the platform (Figure 9-7). The wire is pulled in a horizontal plane (long axis of the platform parallel to the millimeter scale) to permit the proper length of the prosthesis to ensure proper fit (4.5 and 4.25 mm). Over 90 percent of cases use 4.5-mm prostheses (the distance between the footplate and the upper surface of the long crus of the incus).

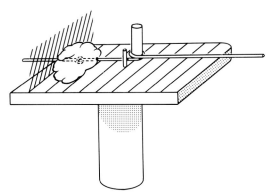

Figure 9-7

The wire is carefully turned approximately 90° against the small post in a counterclockwise direction thus leaving the fatty tissue end of the prosthesis (left-hand side in Figure 9-8) perpendicular to the free end (right-hand side in Figure 9-8) of the prosthesis.

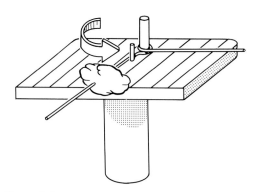

Figure 9-8

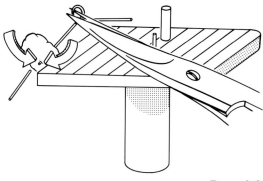

Figure 9-9

A knife blade may be used to elevate the prosthesis from the die platform. Wire cutters are used to open the loop close to the long shaft. Keeping the cutters balanced on the platform should minimize all unsteady motions (Figure 9-9). Alligator forceps may be used to open the loop about 1 mm. It should fit easily on the long post (the same size as the long crus of the incus). The shaft beyond the fatty tissue is snipped off. Keeping the cutters against the fatty tissue will ensure that the prosthesis does not shoot off the table.

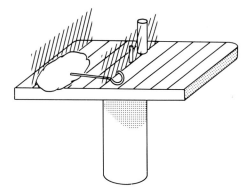

Figure 9-10

Measurement of the prosthesis length is again made, and if several prostheses are made, they are carefully placed in separate cups on the scrub table (Figure 9-10). The prosthesis is kept in saline or Ringer's solution until it is ready for placement.

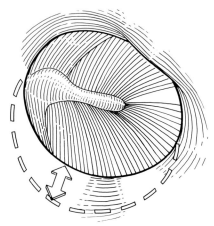

Figure 9-11

A standard stapedectomy incision is made starting from the 12 o'clock position to the 6 o'clock position in a curvilinear fashion (Figure 9-11). The widest diameter from the annulus should be approximately 6 mm. The House lancet or oval knife can be used. Superiorly, firm pressure is needed to cut through the fibrous tissues.

The elevation of the tympanomeatal flap can be done with a small cotton ball attached to the No. 5 suction tip (Figure 9-12). The cotton ball should be first moistened with 1% lidocaine with epinephrine. This method is particularly useful when oozing is encountered.

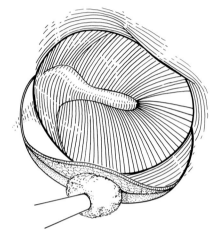

Figure 9-12

The elevation can also be done bimanually with simultaneous suctioning (Figure 9-13). The No. 3 or 20 suction tip should be used. Note that the suction tip shown in Figure 9-13 is placed just in front of the elevator knife to prevent tearing of the flap by excessive suction.

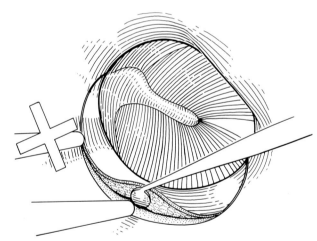

Figure 9-13

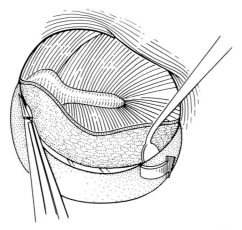

The Bellucci alligator scissors is very useful in completing the incision at the upper and lower ends. The annulus tympanicus should be carefully identified and gently elevated (Figure 9-14).

Figure 9-14

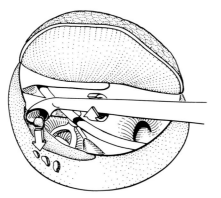

Using House sharp stapes curet (K or J curet), the surgeon curets the posterosuperior bony rim away until the pyramidal eminence or the posterior portion of the footplate becomes easily visible (Figure 9-15). Sweeping strokes should be employed and directed laterally away from the incus. The chorda tympani should be carefully identified and pushed forward before the bony rim is curetted.

Figure 9-15

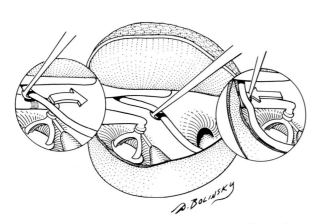

Following satisfactory visualization of the tympanic space, the chorda tympani is often lying in the midportion of the operating field (Figure 9-16). Gentle mobilization of the chorda tympani nerve in its anterior position will loosen fibrous attachments to the manubrium. The chorda may then be stretched in an inferior direction. Alternatively, following the curetting of the bony rim bone in the superior-posterior region, the chorda may be repositioned in that area to avoid interference with the operative field. Note (in Figure 9-16) that work on the nerve is done in the anterior portion where tension is avoided in the region of the iter chordae posterius.

Figure 9-16

Once satisfactory visualization of the operative field has been obtained, the surgeon should demonstrate ossicular mobility in case, in addition to stapes fixation, the malleus and/or incus is fixed. As shown in Figure 9-17, traction is placed on the undersurface of the manubrium and the malleus mobility is demonstrated. Furthermore, gentle traction on the long process of the incus will demonstrate its mobility about the incudostapedial joint. Finally, to make the diagnosis of otosclerosis, the stapes suprastructure is *gently* manipulated in a superior-inferior direction without disarticulating the suprastructure from the remaining ossicular chain.

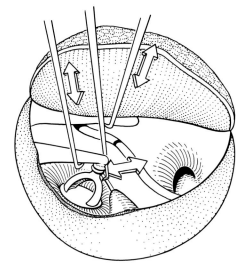

Figure 9-17

Once stapes fixation is established, a measuring rod is used (Figure 9-18). The surgeon must use either a House measuring instrument that goes to the upper surface of the long process of the incus or a Schuknecht instrument that measures the height from the footplate to the *under surface* of the long process of the incus. Note the insert to Figure 9-18, which shows the relative positioning of both the House and Schuknecht measuring instruments in relationship to the long process of the incus and the stapes footplate.

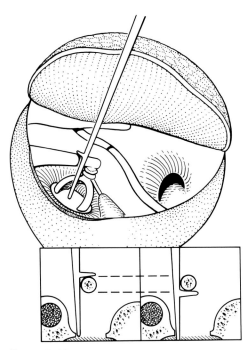

Figure 9-18

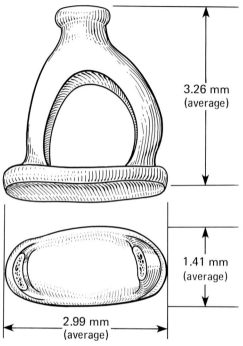

3.26 mm
(average)

1.41 mm
(average)

2.99 mm
(average)

Figure 9-19

Prior to the mobilization and separation of the stapes suprastructure from the footplate, the surgeon should be prepared to use either prefabricated stapes prosthesis or a prosthesis made of autogenous material. In either case, a familiarity with the anatomic size of the average stapes is imperative. Figure 9-19 gives relative sizes of the stapes suprastructure and footplate as determined by Anson and Donaldson.[1] The average height from the capitulum of the stapes to the footplate is 3.26 mm, with a range of 2.56–3.78 mm. The average width of the stapes footplate is 1.41 mm, with a range of 1.08–1.66 mm; the average length of the footplate is 2.99 mm, with a range of 2.64–3.36 mm.

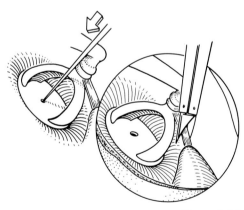

Figure 9-20

Once measured, a fine needle is used to perforate the footplate (Figure 9-20). This maneuver will minimize the chance for a floating footplate. The stapedius tendon is then divided close to the pyramidal eminence to avoid obscuring the footplate region.

The incudostapedial joint is separated cleanly. Note that the joint shown in Figure 9-21 invariably lies in a position more medial than that expected by the novice surgeon. Gentle palpation of this joint may be appreciated by mobilizing the incus in a slightly lateral direction as the incudostapedial joint knife is placed between the lenticular process of the incus and the capitulum of the stapes. Direct trauma to the lenticular process by lateral placement of the knife may traumatize the ossicular chain.

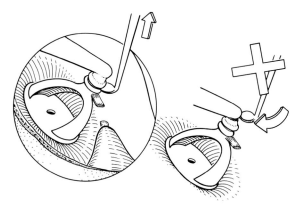

Figure 9-21

In a smooth steady motion, the stapes suprastructure is rocked toward the promontory. (Figure 9-22). The fewer number of motions used, the less trauma delivered to the footplate and, in turn, the inner ear.

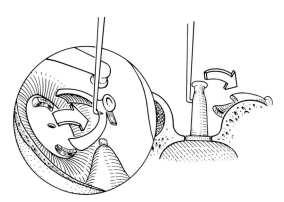

Figure 9-22

The stapes is grasped with a cup forceps and removed (Figure 9-23). If the ossicle is dislodged into the hypotympanum or sinus tympani region, minimal effort should be employed in retrieving it as its presence in the tympanic space is benign.

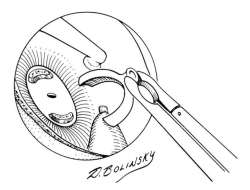

Figure 9-23

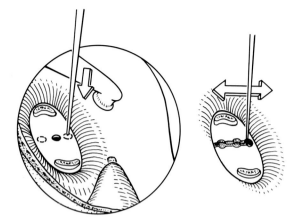

The footplate is gently scored in the central region, thus fracturing it into two pieces (Figure 9-24).

Figure 9-24

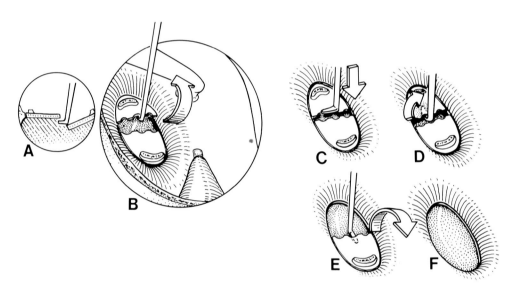

Figure 9-25

A Hough hoe (90°) is introduced, depressing the central limb of the posterior fragment (Figure 9-25A) and elevating the anterior fragment (Figure 9-25B). Alternatively, the Hough hoe is placed between the two fragments with its long axis parallel to the bisected ends of the footplate (Figure 9-25C). The hoe is then turned 90° and the anterior segment is removed (Figure 9-25D). Subsequently, the posterior fragment is removed (Figure 9-25E). From the time the footplate is exposed and the vestibule opened, the surgeon should use only a No. 24 suction, and not in the vicinity of the vestibule (Figure 9-25F).

In Figure 9-26 the prosthesis is grasped with a toothed alligator forceps parallel to the shaft. The crook should not be directly grasped, thus avoiding altering its shape. The loop is carefully placed over the long process of the incus.

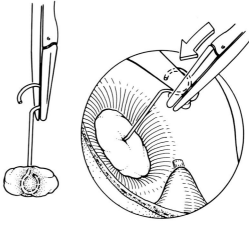

Figure 9-26

Once positioned (both about the long process of the incus and within the oval window), the wire is crimped evenly by closing the instrument in an anterior-to-posterior direction (Figure 9-27). No movement other than the circumferential crimping should be employed.

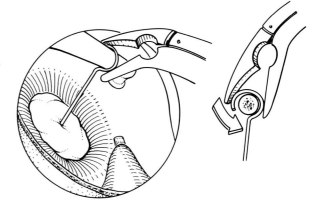

Figure 9-27

The tympanomeatal flap is placed in position and the canal packed (Figure 9-28).

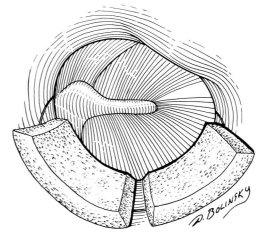

Figure 9-28

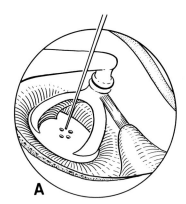

A

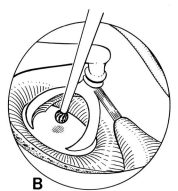

B

Figure 9-29

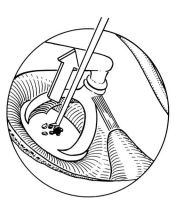

Figure 9-30

ALTERNATIVE PROCEDURES

Small-Fenestra Stapedectomy (Stapedotomy)

Stapedotomy is a useful recommended procedure for advanced otosclerosis with a completely fixed, thick-stapes footplate. Although it has several advantages over stapedectomy, it is more difficult to perform for early otosclerosis with minimally fixed footplate.

One advantage of a stapedotomy is that a small fenestra through the stapes footplate carries much less risk of inner ear injury. There are fibrous adhesions between the superior portion of the footplate and the utricle present in two-thirds of the temporal bones studied by Fisch.[5] Total removal of the footplate, therefore, may damage the inner ear membranes. Stapedotomy also provides better stability for the prosthesis and decreases the risk of postoperative fistula formation. Stapedotomy performs significantly better than stapedectomy at 4 kHz, but the hearing result at 0.5–2 kHz is slightly poorer than after stapedectomy.[5]

Preparation and entrance into the middle-ear space is performed in a fashion similar to that described for total stapedectomy. With otosclerosis defined by use of a fine needle, perforations of the footplate may define the perimeter of a 0.8–1.0-mm fenestration of the oval window (Figure 9-29A). Alternatively, a fenestra of the same size may be obtained with cautious drilling as demonstrated in Figure 9-29B.

Following the fenestration of the oval window, a 1-mm 90° hook may be carefully inserted to remove a small fragment of the footplate (Figure 9-30).

The stapedial tendon is divided close to the pyramidal eminence (Figure 9-31).

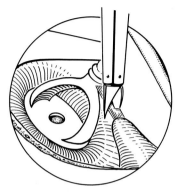

Figure 9-31

The incudostapedial joint is carefully separated (Figure 9-32). Placement of the joint knife should be done in such a fashion that trauma to the lenticular process does not occur.

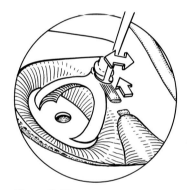

Figure 9-32

The suprastructure of the stapes is removed after separation from the footplate with either crurotomy scissors or with an incudostapedial joint knife (Figure 9-33).

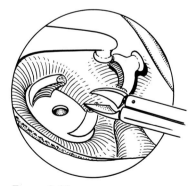

Figure 9-33

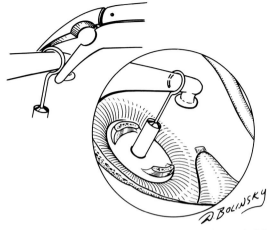

Figure 9-34

Following the removal of the suprastructure, the Teflon wire piston is placed (Figure 9-34). Note that the wire is crimped evenly by closing the instrument in an anterior to posterior direction. No movement other than the circumferential crimping should be employed. Alternatively, Fisch has recently described the small fenestra stapedotomy technique employing the placement of the piston, following fenestration, prior to the disarticulation and removal of the stapes suprastructure.

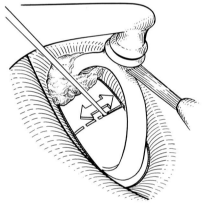

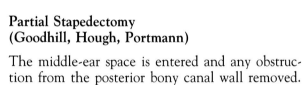

Figure 9-35

Partial Stapedectomy
(Goodhill, Hough, Portmann)

The middle-ear space is entered and any obstruction from the posterior bony canal wall removed. The footplate is scored with a fine chisel or needle and smoothly fractured. This will decompress the vestibule and permit mobilization of the footplate fragment (Figure 9-35).

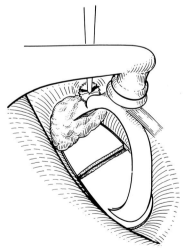

Figure 9-36

The anterior crura limb is separated from the stapes suprastructure (Figure 9-36).

The anterior footplate fragment along with the focus of otosclerotic bone is removed. The posterior fragment shown in Figure 9-37 is maintained in position. Some otologists mobilize the posterior fragment by displacing it toward the promontory,[8] whereas others separate the crura and rotate the suprastructure.[15]

Autogenous graft material (vein or perichondrium) is placed in the oval window niche as the suprastructure is "reflected" anteriorly (Figure 9-38A). The posterior arch and attendent footplate is repositioned over the graft (Figure 9-38B). This delicate manipulation of the suprastructure is quite a difficult task, and this technique may not be the optimal choice in stapes surgery for the inexperienced surgeon.

Laser Stapedectomy (Perkins)

In 1980 Perkins[14] advocated the use of argon laser (*not carbon dioxide*) for stapedectomy. Although this technique has significant advantages, such as ease of crurotomy and precise footplate fenestration, we caution the general otologist that certain characteristics of the argon laser have not yet been proved safe for the patient. The unpredictable combination of footplate thickness, lack of pigmentation in the bone, transmission of the laser beam through the bone, and degree of mineralization is compounded in patients with otosclerosis. While the final layer of bone is vaporized, the laser beam may penetrate deeply, causing the inner ear damage. Animal experiments by Gantz et al.[7] showed saccular membrane fistula in 37 percent of ears examined following argon laser stapedectomy.

Following the elevation of the tympanomeatal flap and the removal of the posterosuperior bony canal wall, the ossicular chain is evaluated as in traditional stapes surgery (Figure 9-39). After the diagnosis is made, the stapedial tendon is vaporized. Multiple pulses (100 msec/per 0.5–0.8 W) are employed. A suction (No. 24) will aid in keeping the field free of vapors.

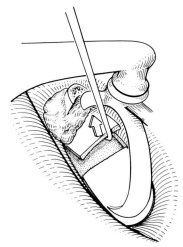

Figure 9-37

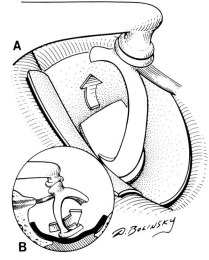

Figure 9-38

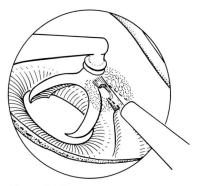

Figure 9-39

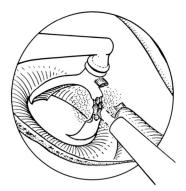

Figure 9-40

The posterior crus is vaporized (Figure 9-40).

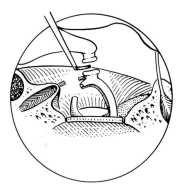

Figure 9-41

The incudostapedial joint is separated and the suprastructure fractured toward the promontory (Figure 9-41).

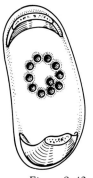

Figure 9-42

A stapedotomy hole is outlined in rosette fashion (Figure 9-42). The focal spot (50–100 μm) is used at 0.4–0.7 W per 100-msec burst. The size of the stapedotomy should reflect the diameter of the planned prosthesis. The outline should be conservatively done over several minutes to minimize thermal trauma to the vestibule.

A fine 45° pick is used to elevate the footplate (Figure 9-43).

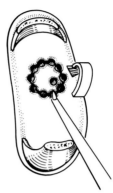

Figure 9-43

Completed stapedotomy is shown in Figure 9-44.

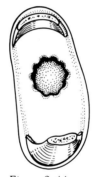

Figure 9-44

Placement of the piston with vein graft is shown in Figure 9-45.

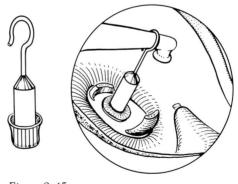

Figure 9-45

SELECTION OF PROSTHESIS

Since the introduction of polyethylene strut for sta-pedial prosthesis by Shea,[20] many different prostheses have been developed (Figure 9-46). The author still prefers the fat-wire prosthesis for both total and small-fenestra stapedectomy.

Prostheses developed for this purpose include the Shea vein—polyethylene strut (Figure 9-46A), Schuknecht fat-wire prosthesis (B), House wire prosthesis on compressed Gelfoam (C), Schuk-necht Gelfoam-wire prosthesis (D), Armstrong modification of Schuknecht Gelfoam-wire pros-thesis with large wire loop and tapered Gelfoam (E), Robinson stainless steel piston (F), Shea Tef-lon cup piston (G), Shea stainless steel prosthesis (H), McGee stainless steel prosthesis (I), Teflon wire piston (J), Sheehy incus replacement pros-thesis (K), and Schuknecht Teflon wire malleus attachment prosthesis (L), fat-wire piston, (M).

For stapedotomy cases, the author uses a "fat-wire piston." The fat-wire prosthesis is first made in the usual fashion, and then the fat is trimmed, leaving a minimal amount of fat (shaped like a piston) to fit the small fenestra (Figure 9-46M).

STAPEDECTOMY IN FENESTRATED EAR

Shambaugh[19] states: "A stapedectomy in an ear unsuccessfully fenestrated in the first place is doomed to failure if the initial failure was due to serous labyrinthitis, and such an ear is very vulnerable to further hearing loss by surgery that opens the laby-rinth."

Sheehy has noted that surgery for a patient who has had a fenestration is contraindicated if there is a history of no hearing gain following fenestration with an air-bone gap of 40 dB or greater.[22]

The young otologist should note that this is a tech-nically difficult procedure and should practice on the temporal bone specimen first many times before undertaking this on the patient. The otologist should learn to crimp the upper loop of the wire prosthesis around the manubrium without leaving an open space; otherwise, the entire wire prosthesis may be found extruding into the ear canal a few years later.

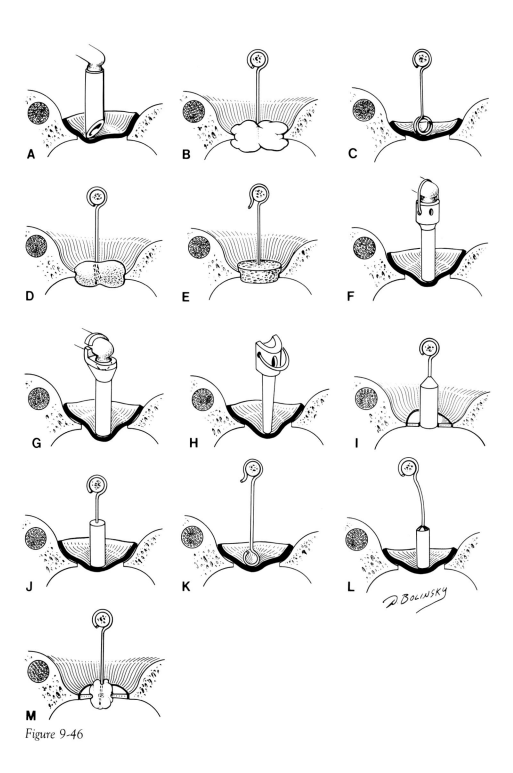

Figure 9-46

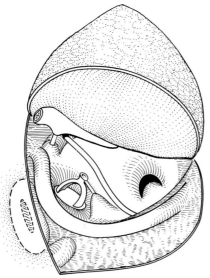

Figure 9-47

MALLEUS TO OVAL WINDOW FAT-WIRE PROSTHESIS TECHNIQUE (SCHUKNECHT)

The fenestration cavity is carefully examined. In Figure 9-47, note the absence of the incus and the head of the malleus following initial fenestration surgery. The cavity is gently debrided of all squamous material, and the thin posterior canal wall skin overlying the horizontal canal is appreciated. The initial fenestra on the horizontal semicircular canal may or may not be recognizable. The tympanomeatal flap is elevated anterior to the horizontal canal and posterolaterally to the facial nerve, exposing the tympanic space.

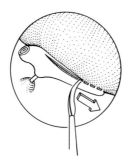

Figure 9-48

With the use of a sickle knife, a horizontal incision is made on the posterolateral aspect of the manubrium, and the tympanic membrane is carefully teased off the manubrium along its lateral surface (Figure 9-48). The drum should not be torn during its elevation.

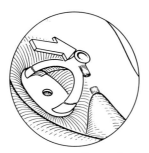

Figure 9-49

Classic stapes suprastructure disarticulation is performed (Figure 9-49).

A fat-wire prosthesis is constructed (Figure 9-50) (see also Figures 9-5–10). Remember that the distance from the malleus to the footplate will range from 5 to 7.25 mm, with an average of 6.25 mm.

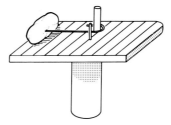

Figure 9-50

The prosthesis wire is carefully placed about the manubrium with its crook and shaft lying perpendicular to the long axis of the manubrium (Figure 9-51).

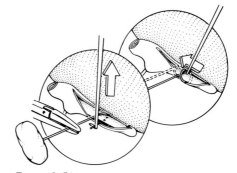

Figure 9-51

The fat-wire prosthesis is gently placed into the oval window niche having a smooth curve along the shaft (Figure 9-52). The crook must be crimped about the circumference of the manubrium without folding on itself or leaving any "open space." This will prevent later extrusion of the wire prosthesis.

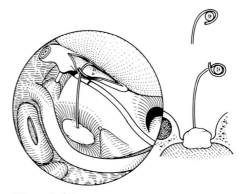

Figure 9-52

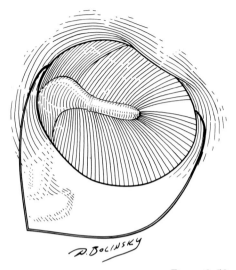

Figure 9-53

The drum is replaced in its anatomic position and the canal packed (Figure 9-53).

ALTERNATIVE PROCEDURES

Incus Replacement Prosthesis (IRP) Technique (Sheehy)

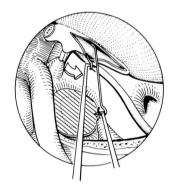

Figure 9-54

The IRP shown in Figure 9-54 has been looped around the manubrium of the malleus and is being guided down onto an autogenous covering over the oval window. Note the careful bimanual manipulation to ensure that the crook of the incus replacement prosthesis wire completely circumscribes the manubrium. In Sheehy's experience, a 5.75-mm IRP has been the proper length in most nonfenestrated ears. In fenestrated ears the usual reported length has been 5.25–5.5 mm.

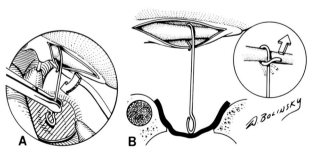

Figure 9-55

As shown in Figure 9-55A, the prosthesis has been crimped about the manubrium by gentle direct wire crimping as opposed to the standard circumferential anterior-to-posterior crimping usually employed for stapedectomy prosthesis placements. The distal end of the wire is juxtaposed against the graft over the oval window. Figure 9-55B is an artist's view of the position of the incus replacement prosthesis. Gelfoam is generally placed about the prosthesis to prevent mobilization in the postoperative period.

Transtympanic Prosthesis Technique (Sheer)

The fenestration cavity is prepared, and a tympanomeatal flap is elevated (Figure 9-56). A traditional stapedectomy is performed. The tympanic membrane is reflected back into its anatomic position by using a sharp pick or a sickle knife. Score holes in the drum midway between the umbo and the short process of the malleus are made immediately next to the manubrium. The posterior perforation is enlarged and the prosthesis (Polytef wire with oversized loop) is introduced.

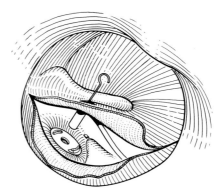

Figure 9-56

Placement is accomplished by alternating position between intratympanic and extratympanic manipulation (Figure 9-57). The prosthesis is crimped externally. The proper looping of the ossicle by the crimper may be determined by intratympanic inspection. The drum is placed back in its anatomic position, and the iatrogenic perforations can be expected to close within 2 weeks.

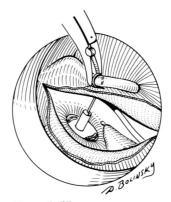

Figure 9-57

TORP and Cartilage Technique (Fisch)

The fenestration cavity is prepared, and a tympanomeatal flap is elevated (Figure 9-58A). A subtotal stapedectomy is performed. The footplate is covered with autogenous graft material (perichondrium), and a TORP is placed. Note that the chorda tympani shown in Figure 9-58A is used to support the graft. Cartilage (septal) is placed lateral to the TORP, and the tympanomeatal flap is returned (Figure 9-58B).

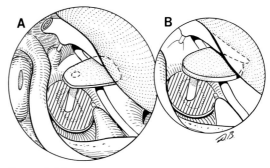

Figure 9-58

PROBLEMS AND SOLUTIONS DURING SURGERY

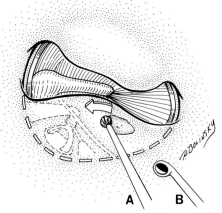

Figure 9-59

NARROW EAR CANAL

For cartilaginous or bony canal obstructions, ear canalplasty and/or a meatoplasty should be done as the first procedure. At times, one may encounter excessive bony overhang of the posterosuperior canal wall near the annulus tympanicus. This bony exostoses can be removed by a drill (Figure 9-59A) or curet (Figure 9-59B) until the entire stapes becomes visible.

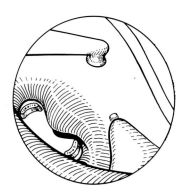

Figure 9-60

NARROW OVAL WINDOW NICHE

The inferior margin and the oval window membrane are obstructed by a bony overhang (Figure 9-60). Changes in the size of the oval window niche and/or stapes may indicate a congenital malformation.

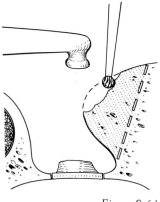

Figure 9-61

The bony obstruction is burred down with a saucerization technique from lateral to medial (Figure 9-61). The operator must avoid drilling into a "hole." Cognizance of the vestibular location of the saccule and utricle must be kept in mind.

Prior to removal of the footplate, all bony fragments must be evacuated to avoid contamination of the labyrinth. The prosthesis is then placed (Figure 9-62).

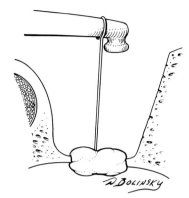

Figure 9-62

FLOATING FOOTPLATE

Schuknecht notes that previous stapes mobilization and minimal footplate fixation are the two conditions that most often lead to a floating footplate.

Occasionally a 1-mm right-angle hook may be able to direct the fragment against the wall of the niche and the bone may be elevated out of the oval window (Figure 9-63).

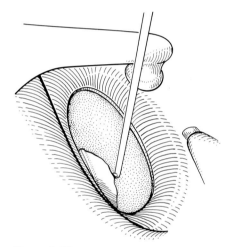

Figure 9-63

The suction is placed *lateral* to the elevated fragments (Figure 9-64). Suction should *not* be applied to the vicinity of the open window. Bimanual manipulation may effect removal.

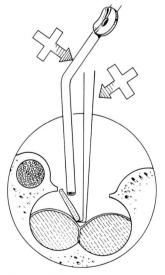

Figure 9-64

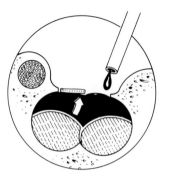

Figure 9-65

Blood is placed in the vestibule[23] in an attempt to float the bony fragment (Figure 9-65).

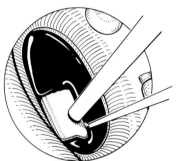

Figure 9-66

In Figure 9-66 the fragment is seen floating on the coagulum of blood. Note the flush juxtaposition of the suction on the fragment. This will avoid a "dry hole."

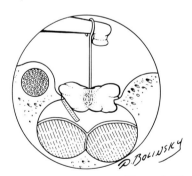

Figure 9-67

Usually the fragment can be retrieved. If stabilized, the prosthesis is placed atraumatically and buttressed against the fragment (Figure 9-67).

Note: On rare occasion, a fragment of instrument may break off and displace into the oval window following removal of the footplate. If the fragment is deep in the vestibule, however, it is *best left undisturbed.*

DEPRESSED FRAGMENTS

At times this complication may not be amenable to intraoperative rectification. The inexperienced surgeon is cautioned that manipulation of the vestibule, even of limited extent, is associated with both dysequilibrium and potential sensorineural hearing loss.

The footplate is uniformly depressed following suprastructure removal (Figure 9-68). A 1-mm sharp hook engages the anterior crural stump and elevation laterally is performed.

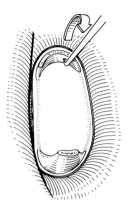

Figure 9-68

The posterior crural stump is stabilized while a fine hook (45° or 90°) is inserted parallel to the long axis of the footplate and rotated 90° (Figure 9-69). Elevation is cautiously attempted.

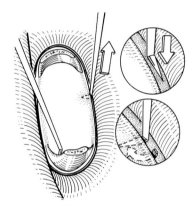

Figure 9-69

Schuknecht recommends using a 0.5-mm sharp cutting burr to notch the inferior wall of the oval window. A 0.3-mm hook is introduced, and the depressed footplate is mobilized laterally (Figure 9-70).

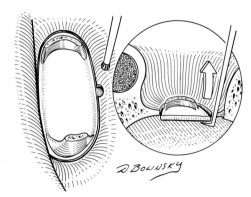

Figure 9-70

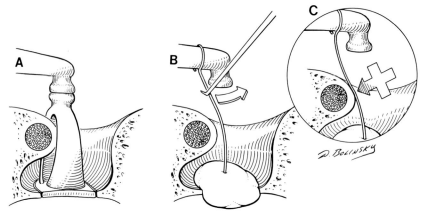

Figure 9-71

ABNORMAL FACIAL NERVE

The dehiscent facial nerve is not a contraindication to stapes surgery. However, it should caution the surgeon to proceed with utmost care. Furthermore, variable dehiscence of the fallopian canal can occur, and the stapes surgeon should palpate the nerve before undertaking a stapedectomy.

In Figure 9-71A the fallopian canal is noted to overlie the footplate. In Figure 9-71B the suprastructure and footplate bone have been successfully removed. The prosthesis (fat-wire) is placed with a slight bend to the shaft. The wire shown in Figure 9-71C rests on a nondehiscent portion of the fallopian canal. This should be avoided. Mobility of the chain is ensured prior to closing.

OBLITERATED OTOSCLEROSIS

At surgery otosclerosis may be found to obliterate the footplate, and extend into the vestibule. Schuknecht cautions that it may be prudent in these cases to discontinue drilling rather than risk damage to the inner ear.[18]

The oval window is obliterated (Figure 9-72). When drilling begins, the rotation of the drill should favor a protected stroke for the facial nerve.

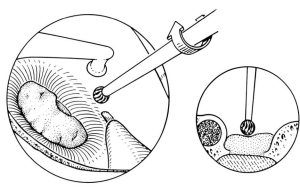

Figure 9-72

The window is saucerized without drilling into a "hole" (Figure 9-73).

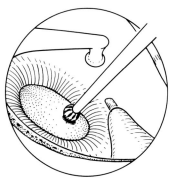
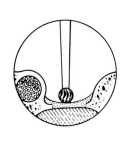

Figure 9-73

A stapedotomy (0.6–1 mm) is performed and the small fragment of bone removed (Figure 9-74).

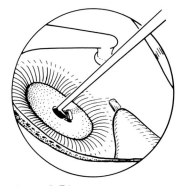
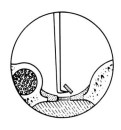

Figure 9-74

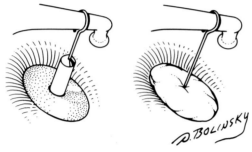

Figure 9-75

A Teflon wire piston is placed with or without autogenous grafting (Figure 9-75). If a large piece of footplate is removed, a fat-wire prosthesis may be placed.

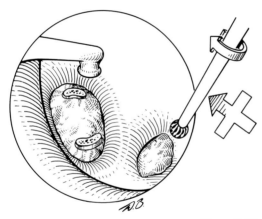

Figure 9-76

ROUND-WINDOW OTOSCLEROSIS

Any surgeon who is not fully convinced that the round window is completely obliterated should proceed with the stapedectomy. Drilling about the round-window niche may provoke a sensorineural hearing loss and should not be done.

As shown in Figure 9-76, both windows are obliterated and stapedectomy will be of little value.

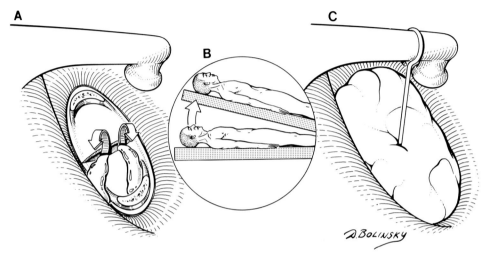

Figure 9-77

CEREBROSPINAL FLUID LEAK

The so-called gusher is an uncommon but nevertheless unsettling intraoperative problem. Its presence is more common in the ear with a congenitally fixed stapes (Schuknecht).

Opening into the vestibule may produce a flow of clear fluid, initially perilymph, and then continued cerebrospinal fluid (CSF) (Figure 9-77A). The patient's head should be elevated above the phlebostatic axis to decrease pressure (Figure 9-77B). *Note:* The patient should be maintained in a head-up position for several days postoperatively. A large fat-wire prosthesis is placed in the oval window as quickly as possible (Figure 9-77C).

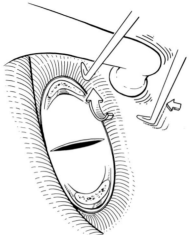

Figure 9-78

INCUS DISLOCATION

Subluxation

For the young surgeon, mobilization of the foot-plate and stapes suprastructure may be so mind oc-cupying that when the stapes is vigorously re-moved, the incus may be traumatized (Figure 9-78). The surgeon should learn how to move the instrument slowly and carefully.

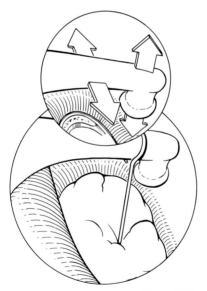

Figure 9-79

Prior to placement of the prosthesis, the incus should be palpated and its mobility appreciated (especially excessive mobility) (Figure 9-79). If the incus is subluxed but moves with the malleus, the pros-thesis should be placed on the incus in the usual manner.

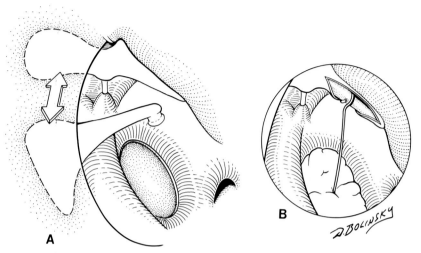

Figure 9-80

Luxation

If the incus has been detached from the malleus, it should be removed (Figure 9-80A). In such a case, a malleus-to-oval window fat-wire prosthesis should be placed (Figure 9-80B) (see also Figures 9-47–9-53).

BLEEDING

Fundamental to safe middle-ear surgery is a dry field. Careful instillation of local anesthetic (Xylocaine with epinephrine) of concentration dilutions that can safely be tolerated by the patient (1:10,000–1:100,000) will at most times afford good visualization. Bleeding, however, may come from an aberrant stapedial artery, middle-ear mucosa, or highly vascularized otosclerotic bone.

Figure 9-81 shows careful instillation of local anesthetic prior to flap elevation.

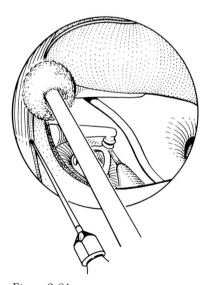

Figure 9-81

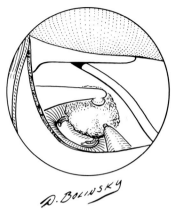

If bleeding is encountered once the ear is opened, epinephrine on a cotton pledget should be applied and the pledget removed (Figure 9-82). Bovie cautery may damage the facial nerve and is not recommended.

Figure 9-82

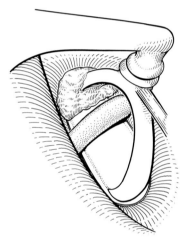

PERSISTENT STAPEDIAL ARTERY

In rare cases the stapedial artery will persist (second arch remnant, Figure 9-83).

Figure 9-83

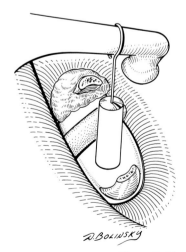

A careful stapedotomy with piston prosthesis may be done (Figure 9-84).

Figure 9-84

MALLEUS FIXATION
(SEE CHAPTER 6)

Failure to recognize malleus fixation will result in anatomically successful, but functionally fruitless stapedectomy, subjecting the patient to another otherwise avoidable operation. It is imperative for the surgeon to check the mobility of all three ossicles at the time of the stapedectomy.

For management of malleus fixation, please refer to Chapter 6, on ossicular reconstruction.

TEAR OF
TYMPANOMEATAL FLAP

Small rents in the canal wall skin may be left to heal; however, a tear in the drum should be repaired. Generally this may be done with a small plug of fat obtained from the lobule.

The margins of the small perforation are elevated and approximated (Figure 9-85).

Fat is placed through the rent or under the tympanomeatal flap to be medial to the tear; perichondrium or fascia may be used (Figure 9-86).

The flap is returned, and a portion of the graft is appreciated to occlude the perforation (Figure 9-87).

PROBLEMS AND
SOLUTIONS AFTER
SURGERY

REPARATIVE GRANULOMA

There exist few emergencies encountered by the otologic surgeon. Recognition and treatment of this clinical problem, however, is one of them.

The clinical picture includes (1) vague constitutional symptoms 1–2 weeks following surgery; (2) decreased hearing following an initial gain along with decreased discrimination; (3) dysequilibrium; (4) aural fullness; and (5) dull red, thickened hy-

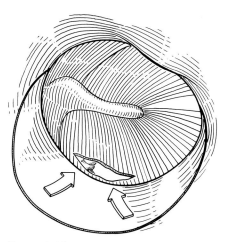

Figure 9-85

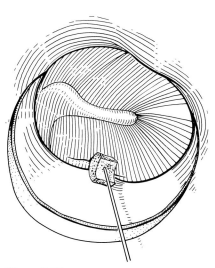

Figure 9-86

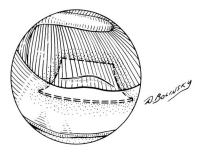

Figure 9-87

pervascular skin flap with inflammation in the posterosuperior quadrant of the tympanic membrane. The audiometric test will show a mixed and/or sensorineural hearing loss (especially in high frequencies) and decreased discrimination.

Treatment consists of complete removal of the granuloma and prosthesis, and replacement of the new fat-wire prosthesis.

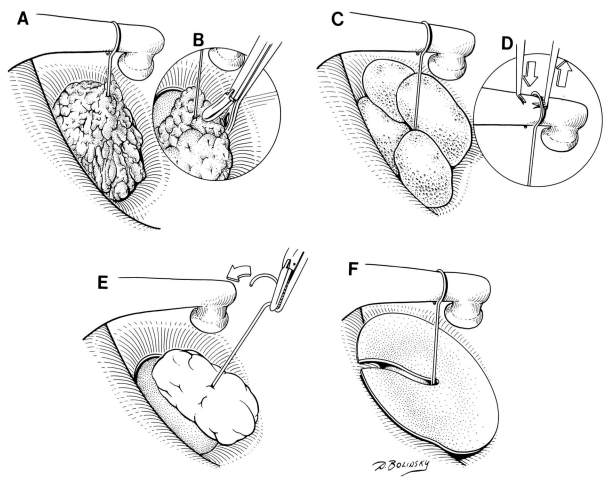

Figure 9-88

Granuloma may envelope the oval window and the prosthesis as shown in Figure 9-88A. It may involve the vestibule, the incus, and rarely the entire middle-ear space. The granuloma is removed piecemeal with a cup forceps (Figure 9-88B). Gelfoam soaked with Xylocaine and epinephrine is placed for hemostasis (Figure 9-88C). The prosthesis is lifted carefully off the incus by gentle pressure as depicted in Figure 9-88D. A new prosthesis is fashioned (Figure 9-88E). A fascia covering is placed over the new graft (Figure 9-88F). According to Schuknecht granulomas have not been shown to recur.

PERILYMPH FISTULA

Early postoperative trauma (direct or barotrauma) may displace the prosthesis, leading to a perilymph fistula. Delayed fistulae do occur and must be considered in symptomatic patients.

Central Fistula

A Teflon-wire prosthesis with a periprosthetic leak is shown in Figure 9-89.

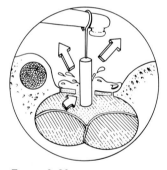

Figure 9-89

The tube is shown in Figure 9-90 acting as a conduit for the fistulous discharge.

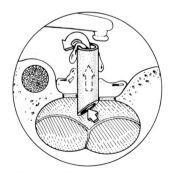

Figure 9-90

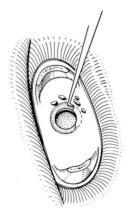

Margins of the fenestra are cleaned following removal of the prosthesis (Figure 9-91).

Figure 9-91

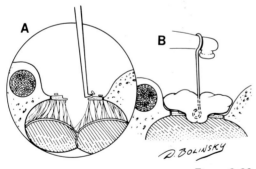

In Figure 9-92A note the fibrous adhesions to the
undersurface of the oval window membrane. These
should not be disturbed. A fat-wire prosthesis is
placed as shown in Figure 9-92B.

Figure 9-92

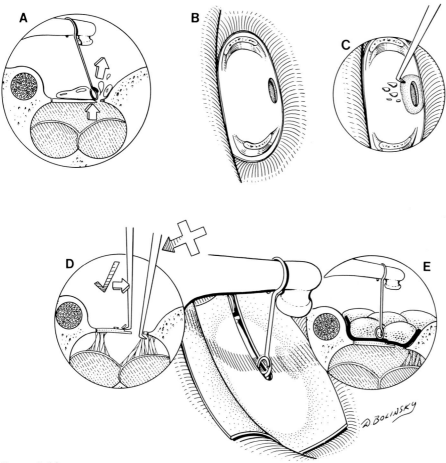

Figure 9-93

Peripheral Fistula

The prosthesis shown in Figure 9-93A has been disrupted and migrated to the inferior pole of the oval window with a perilymph leak. The prosthesis is removed (Figure 9-93B). The upper side of the membrane overlying the window is carefully prepared for regrafting (Figure 9-93C). In Figure 9-93D note that instrumentation should be done at the level of the bony margins, and not below. This will avoid disruption of fibrous adhesions that are present within the vestibule. A fascia graft is placed over the fistula and oval window and a wire prosthesis is placed (Figure 9-93E).

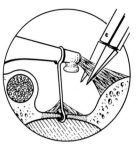

Figure 9-94

FIBROSIS

Fibrosis rarely occurs about the footplate. More commonly, it is found about the incus.

Fibrous adhesive bonds from the incus to the promontory are sharply incised without traumatizing the middle ear or prosthesis (Figure 9-94).

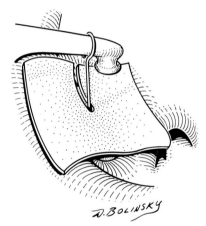

Figure 9-95

Gelfilm or silastic is placed to prevent fibrous band reformation (Figure 9-95).

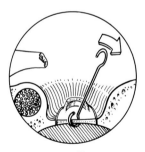

Figure 9-96

INCUS NECROSIS

Resorption of the long process of the incus appears to be caused by either direct surgical trauma or irritation from the prosthesis. There appears to be no scientific basis for the concept of ischemic necrosis due to a tight loop (Schuknecht).[18]

The long process of the incus has been disrupted with the separation of the lateral portion of the graft wire (Figure 9-96).

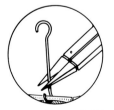

Figure 9-97

The wire may be clipped off and then the malleus-to-oval window prosthesis applied (Figure 9-97).

An alternative approach is to leave the original displaced prosthesis and apply a malleus-to-oval window prosthesis (Figure 9-98).

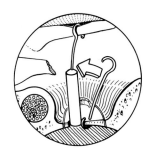

Figure 9-98

After the new prosthesis is in position, the displaced wire is attached to the new prosthesis as shown in Figure 9-99.

Note that the new prosthesis rests on the oval window membrane, and *does not* enter the vestibule.

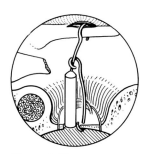

Figure 9-99

Use of the incus homograft as a columella strut is demonstrated in Figure 9-100.

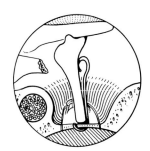

Figure 9-100

Use of a TORP is shown in Figure 9-101. Cartilage is placed lateral to the TORP below the tympanic membrane.

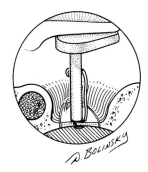

Figure 9-101

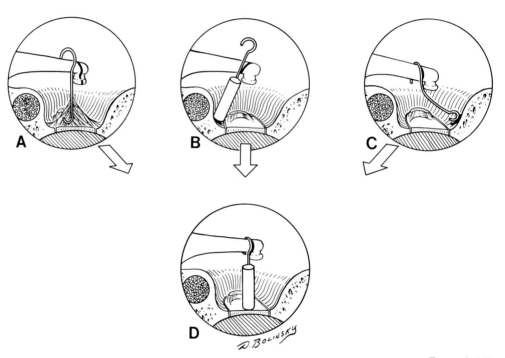

Figure 9-102

DISPLACED PROSTHESIS

Figure 9-102A–C shows potential positions of displaced prostheses. The treatment requires replacement of the prosthesis (Figure 9-102D). Note that the prosthesis does not penetrate the oval window membrane.

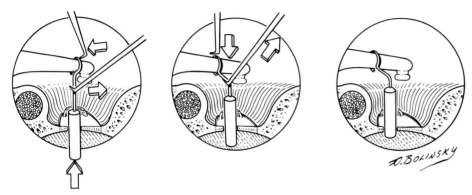

Figure 9-103

A conservative method of correction of a medially displaced Teflon-wire prosthesis is shown in Figure 9-103. Note that the shaft is bent in order to shorten the prosthesis.

REFERENCES

1. Anson, B. J. and Donaldson, J. A.: Surgical Anatomy of the Temporal Bone and Ear. 2nd ed. W.B. Saunders, Philadelphia, 1973.
2. Farrior, B.: Contraindications to the Small Hole Stapedectomy. *Ann. Otol. Rhinol. Laryngol.*, 90:636–639, 1981.
3. Feldman, B. A. and Schuknecht, H. F.: Experiences with Revision Stapedectomy Procedures. *Laryngoscope*, 80:1281–1291, 1970.
4. Fisch, U. P.: Stapedotomy vs Stapedectomy. In: Ear Clinics International, Vol III, Clinical Otology, Paparella, M. M. and Meyerhoff, W. L. (Eds.). Williams & Wilkins, Baltimore, chap. 11, 1983.
5. Fisch, U. P.: Tympanoplasty and Stapedectomy. Thieme-Stratton, New York, 1980.
6. Gacek, R. R.: The Diagnosis and Treatment of Post Stapedectomy Granulomas. *Ann. Otol. Rhinol. Laryngol.*, 79:970–975, 1970.
7. Gantz, B. J., Jenkins, H. A., Kishimoto, S., *et al.*: Argon Laser Stapedectomy. *Ann. Otol. Rhinol. Laryngol.*, 90:25–26, 1982.
8. Goodhill, V.: Posterior Arch Stapedectomy. Ten Commandments for Stapedectomy. *Arch. Otolaryngol.*, 100:460–464, 1974.
9. Hough, J. V. D.: Partial Stapedectomy. *Ann. Otol. Rhinol. Laryngol.*, 69:571, 1960.
10. House, H. P.: The Prefabricated Wire Hoop-Gelfoam Stapedectomy. *Arch. Otolaryngol.*, 76:298–302, 1962.
11. House, H. P., House, W. F., and Hildyard, V. H.: Congenital Stapes Footplate Fixation. *Laryngoscope*, 68:1387, 1958.
12. House, H. P., Linthicum, F. H., and House, J. W.: Stapes Surgery; Footplate Fragmentation in Otosclerosis Surgery. *Laryngoscope*, 80:1256, 1970.
13. McGee, T. M.: Comparison of Small Fenestra and Total Stapedectomy. *Ann. Otol. Rhinol. Laryngol.*, 90:633–636, 1981.
14. Perkins, R. C.: Laser Stapedotomy for Otosclerosis. *Laryngoscope*, 90:228–241, 1980.
15. Portmann, M.: Procedure of Interposition for Otosclerosis deafness. *Laryngoscope*, 70:166–174.
16. Robinson, M.: Total Footplate Extraction in Stapedectomy. *Ann. Otol. Rhinol. Laryngol.*, 90:630–632, 1981.
17. Rosen, S.: Mobilization of the Stapes to Restore Hearing in Otosclerosis. *N.Y. J. Med.*, 53:2650–2653, 1953.
18. Schuknecht, H. F.: *Stapedectomy*. Little, Brown, Boston, 1971.
19. Shambaugh, G. E. and Glasscock, M. E., III, Surgery of the Ear. Ed. 3. W.B. Saunders, Philadelphia, 1980.
20. Shea, J. J., Jr.: Fenestration of the Oval Window. *Ann. Otol. Rhinol. Laryngol.*, 67:932, 1958.
21. Sheehy, J. L. and Powers, W. H.: Incus Replacement Prosthesis in Otosclerotic Surgery. *Arch. Otolaryngol.*, 89:393–398, 1969.
22. Sheehy, J. L., Nelson, R. A., and House, H. P.: Revision Stapedectomy: A Review of 258 Cases. *Laryngoscope*, 91:43–51, 1981.
23. Sheer, A. A.: Retrieving the Lost Heavy Footplate Fragment. *Arch. Otolaryngol.*, 91:412, 1970.
24. Sheer, A. A. and Amjad, A. H.: A New Method of Incus Bypass Stapedectomy. *Arch. Otolaryngol.*, 100:322, 1974.

10
Background Information
on Mastoidectomy

K. J. Lee
Myles L. Pensak

Woven through the fabric of this text is the concept that there exist few, if any, times in medicine when there is only "one correct way" of performing a procedure. Cognizance of this most important point will allow the reader the freedom of intellectual exploration and subsequent prudent choice of technique when preparing for surgery. Incorporation of this principle, a sound knowledge of the pathophysiologic processes involved, and an appreciation of historic trends will eventually lead to both patient and physician satisfaction. Surgery on the mastoid highlights these points and surely reflects the successes, frustrations, and failures of the otologist.

HISTORIC OVERVIEW

Credit for the concept of a mastoid evacuation of disease is given to Ambroise Paré while Jean Petit is cited as the first surgeon to perform the procedure (1736). A succinct review of the history of mastoid surgery is given by Milstein. Table 10-1 outlines some of the significant events leading up to the current era of mastoid surgery.

Table 10-1
Mastoid Surgery: Historic Outline

Date	Physician	
1649	Riolanus	Described mastoid surgery for Eustachian tube dysfunction and tinnitus
1736	Petit	Mastoidectomy
1853	Wilde	Described the postauricular incision for abscess drainage
1873	Schwartze	Described the simple mastoidectomy
1870–1890	Von Tröltsch Zaufal Stacke Von Bergmann	Refined and changed surgical procedures involving mastoid
1885	Kessel	Described endaural approach
1899	Körner	Suggested preservation of tympanic membrane and ossicles under certain circumstances
1910	Bondy	Described modified radical mastoidectomy
1951	Zöllner Wullstein	Tympanoplasty
1950–1960	House Sheehy	Canal wall up procedure

PROCEDURES

CORTICAL (SIMPLE) MASTOIDECTOMY

In this procedure the posterior bony canal wall is completely preserved. The middle ear is not entered. The mastoid is drilled, exposing the antrum, sinodural angle, tegmen, aditus, and mastoid tip cells. Once the emergent procedure for acute suppurative ear infections, this procedure today is indicated for coalescent mastoiditis. Shambaugh[12] notes that the procedure is to be done for the evacuation of purulent material that has been unresponsive to antibiotic therapy and not to prevent chronic otitis media. The air cell system that may be involved pathologically may include the mastoid tip, the root of the zygoma, the sinodural angle, and the periantral and antral cells. The bowl created by the evacuation of diseased cells is bordered by the tegmen, the sinodural angle, the thinned posterior canal wall, and the entrance to the epitympanic space through the antrum.

MODIFIED RADICAL MASTOIDECTOMY (BONDY)

In this operation, the posterior bony canal is taken down. The lateral wall of the epitympanum is removed. The middle ear is not entered. At the conclusion of the procedure, there is an open cavity linking the external auditory canal, epitympanum, antrum, and mastoid. This procedure is usually selected when the middle ear is free of disease and with minimal hearing loss. This exteriorizing technique or the open cavity technique is commonly employed for the removal of cholesteatoma from the attic and mastoid and leaving the matrix as a lining. However, some otologists believe that the matrix, consisting of the squamous and fibrous elements, has been shown to be the source of proteolytic enzymes that are involved in the local tissue destruction. As noted by Abramson,[1] therefore, "the removal of only dead epithelial debris or the leaving of cholesteatoma epithelium behind to line the cavity would not appear to be justified from what we now know of the bone degrading process."

RADICAL MASTOIDECTOMY

This procedure is directed against uncontrolled keratomatous disease involving the mastoid and middle-ear space. One surgical cavity is created, incorporating the mastoid, antrum, epitympanum, tympanum, and external auditory canal. The ossicular chain or the perforated tympanic membrane are not reconstructed. With increasing surgical sophistication and the concomitant prudent usage of local and systemic antibiotics, otologists have come to rely on this operation with less frequency as reconstructive techniques are employed with greater success. The totally open cavity may leave the middle-ear mucosa exposed, leading to weeping and recurrent suppuration.

TYMPANOPLASTY WITH MASTOIDECTOMY

This procedure involves the removal of disease from the mastoid and middle-ear space with immediate or eventual reconstruction of the ossicular chain and tympanic membrane. The surgeon may choose either a "canal wall up" procedure or a "canal wall down" technique. The salient goal of the canal wall up (preservation of the bony posterior canal wall) procedure is to obviate the problems encountered with an open large mastoid cavity. The obliteration technique avoids the disadvantages of a large open cavity and yet affords the wide field approach not available in the "canal wall up" technique. The benefits and potential pitfalls associated with these procedures are discussed.

APPROACHES TO THE MASTOID

Once the decision to perform a mastoidectomy has been made, the surgeon has a choice of approaches to the mastoid.

ENDAURAL APPROACH

This has been described by Lempert, Kessel, Thies Jr., Shambaugh Jr.,[12] House, and Smith.[17] Features of this approach include readily developed meatal flaps, clear exposure of the tympanum, and relative ease of identification of the sinus tympani region (often a difficult site for cholesteatoma evacuation) because the patient may be rotated and the

bony wall taken down over the region without passing through the mastoid. There is also limited exposure to the posterior extension of disease. Hence it is ideal in patients with limited posterior extension of disease. With this approach the formed cavity may also be easily followed and cleaned because the route of surgical access is the same as that to be employed in the followup examinations.

POSTAURICULAR APPROACH

This approach was advocated by Lee and Schuknecht,[7] Paparella, Glasscock, and Sheehy.[13] Features of this approach include direct access to the mastoid, with wide-field approach; ease of harvesting temporalis fascia for tympanic membrane grafting in tympanoplasty associated with mastoidectomy; ready exposure of both zygomatic root, mastoid tip cells, sinodural angle, and tegmen region; amenability to the "canal wall up" procedure; and definition of the sinodural angle in revision surgery as a major landmark.

We recognize that individual skill and training experience play a significant role in determining the procedure employed by the otologist; however, we must emphasize that in our hands, the postauricular incision affords the surgeon the optimal wide field exposure necessary for safe and efficient operating.

The complete removal of disease from the mastoid is considerably dependent on the surgeon's recognition of the pneumatization of the temporal bone and a sound knowledge of where disease is likely to sequester. Allam[3] notes essentially five regions of pneumatization that may serve as locations for pathology: (1) middle-ear space (tympanum, epitympanum, hypotympanum), (2) mastoid, (3) petrous apex, (4) perilabyrinthine spaces, and (5) accessory regions.

The application of this information is reflected in the ablation and cleaning of disease in the following highlighted air-cell tracts:

- Anteroposterior (relative to the eustachian tube)
- Anterolateral (relative to the eustachian tube)
- Hypotympanic
- Retrofacial

- Subarcuate
- Posterosuperior (relative to the endolymphatic sac)
- Posteromedial (relative to the endolymphatic sac)

In spite of this information even the most competent otologic surgeon may become frustrated by the presence of residual or recurrent disease in one of the following regions: facial recess, sinus tympani, mastoid tip, zygomatic root, and sinodural angle.

Kinney[6] recently discussed defensive chronic ear surgery. We feel that a sound knowledge of the potential infection sites is reflected by his comment that "Removal of disease from the ear proceeds in a systematic method. By starting in the same place in every ear and moving step-by-step through the ear, the surgeon is less likely to omit a step. In some cases, the disease has so distorted the ear that we must stop, find a known area, and then move back into the diseased area."*

PROCEDURE HIGHLIGHTS (ANATOMIC FEATURES)

CORTICAL MASTOIDECTOMY

1. Identify the temporal line and create periosteal flaps that permit exposure of the mastoid cortex.
2. Define the spine of Henle; superior and medial to this point is the mastoid antrum.
3. Define the sinodural angle (Citelli's angle).
4. Recognize the presence of Körners septum and avoid identifying a "false antrum."
5. Appreciate the horizontal semicircular canal.
6. Appreciate the lateral portion of the short process of the incus.
7. Saucerize the cavity and thin the posterior canal wall.
8. Thin but do not unroof the bony plate over the sigmoid sinus. Blue lining is not necessary unless the sinus is anteriorly displaced.
9. Ensure that there are no irregular bony edges in the completed bowl.

---

*From Kinney, S.E.: Defensive Chronic Ear Surgery. *Laryngoscope*, 90:1084, 1980. With permission.

MODIFIED RADICAL MASTOIDECTOMY (BONDY)

Follow the design of the cortical mastoidectomy. Take down the bony posterior canal wall. Note that the facial nerve should be medial to the fossa incudi. Then take down the bridge.

Note: Define carefully the facial ridge and note the course of the nerve in its tympanic segment. In the epitympanum the facial nerve lies on the medial wall in the vicinity of the geniculate ganglion. When in doubt, *do not drill.* Use a small stapes curet and direct all strokes laterally—avoiding the facial nerve, horizontal semicircular canal, and dura. A diamond burr drilling in a direction parallel to the facial nerve should be used when approaching the facial ridge.

Use a Körners flap or modification together with obliteration to fill in part of the bowl, cover the inferior portion of the facial ridge, and provide a basis for the epithelization of the bowl. The latter may be done with split-thickness skin grafts.

RADICAL MASTOIDECTOMY

Follow the technique for modified radical. Incorporate the tympanum, with the removal of the tympanic membrane and middle-ear contents, into the created cavity. The stapes should not be disturbed.

FACIAL RECESS APPROACH

This approach is anatomically defined by fossa incudis, facial nerve, and chorda tympani nerve.

In the technique for this approach, posterior canal wall skin is removed in a standard 12:00/6:00 sweep and reflected on an anteroinferior-based pedicule or removed. The ear canal is enlarged, with communication into the mastoid air cell system avoided. The bony anterior canal wall bulge near the annulus is then enlarged, and mastoidectomy is performed. The epitympanum is identified as the wall is taken down in its most posterior superior portion.

Landmarks identified through this approach should include (1) round-window niche, (2) oval-window niche, (3) the horizontal portion of the facial nerve, (4) pyramidal eminence, and (5) cochleariform process.

FACIAL NERVE

Fear of injury to this structure is real and should not be mitigated at any time, even by the most experienced surgeon. However, we feel that the concept that advocates that the safest way to avoid injury is to identify the nerve is correct and should be considered one of the cornerstones of safe, effective surgical technique. Identification of the nerve may be made with the aid of several anatomic structures, as follows:

1. Identify the inferior landmarks: digastric ridge and stylomastoid foramen.
2. Identify the horizontal semicircular canal; the nerve lies anterior and medial at the level of the second genu and inferomedial thereafter.
3. Identify in the middle ear: (a) stapes/oval window, (b) round-window niche, (c) pyramidal process, (d) eustachian tube, and (e) cochleariform process. (This landmark is quite reliable even in the chronic ear with the facial nerve passing just superior and posterior to this process.)
4. Recognize that the proximal horizontal portion of the nerve is located on the medial bony wall of the epitympanum.
5. Identify the incus.
6. Identify the chorda tympani.

COMPLICATIONS OF MASTOID SURGERY

Many of the complications of the disease may be precipitated by complications of the surgery. These include (1) facial nerve injury, (2) increased conductive hearing loss, (3) sensorineural hearing loss, (4) labyrinthitis, (5) perilymph fistulae, (6) dural tear with or without CSF leak, (7) meningitis, (8) abscess—brain or peridural, (9) brain herniation,

(10) lateral sinus hemorrhage, (11) jugular bulb bleeding, (12) venous thrombosis, (13) retained cholesteatoma, (14) mastoid-cutaneous fistulae, and (15) wound infection or continued suppuration.

Discussion persists regarding the wisdom of a closed versus an open cavity as determined by the presence of the "canal wall" being up or down. Since Rambo first reported the obliteration of the mastoid cavity with temporalis muscle in 1958, numerous otologists have reported on the mastoid obliteration procedure. Among them Bartels and Sheehy,[4] Gacek,[5] Lee and Schuknecht,[7] and Palva[9] have all noted certain features of the procedure and given their own recommendations. (*Note:* Realistically, the goal of mastoid cavity obliteration procedure is to make the cavity size smaller and not to completely eliminate the cavity. Together with a large meatus created by meatoplasty, the smaller cavity presents minimal problems.)

OBLITERATION OF THE MASTOID

OBLITERATION TECHNIQUE HIGHLIGHTS (SURGICAL)

First, perform a complete mastoidectomy. Lower the posterior canal wall to the facial ridge. The posterior canal wall skin should be preserved, such as with the use of a Körner flap. The surgical defect is to be filled in with either subcutaneous postauricular tissue and muscle or the more recently described supplemental bone pate. Then the posterior canal wall skin should be placed against the obliteration material.

DISCUSSION

Advantages of the obliteration procedure include rapid healing and minimal postoperative care. Disadvantages include potential to cover residual disease and the potential for reformation of the cavity.

INTACT CANAL WALL

The advantages of the intact canal wall include anatomic preservation of the posterior wall, avoidance of a mastoid cavity that is exteriorized, potential for increased aeration of the middle ear, and tympanic membrane reconstruction occurring in its anatomic position because the tympanic ring is preserved.

Disadvantages of the intact canal wall are that the technique is surgically difficult, it is difficult to expose the attic and sinus tympani regions, and residual disease occurs in even the best of hands. A "second-look" procedure is needed at variable times for residual cholesteatoma and/or ossiculoplasty.

REFERENCES

1. Abramson, M.: Collagenolytic Activity in Middle Ear Cholesteatoma. *Ann. Otol.*, 78:112–125, 1969.
2. Abramson, M. and Gross, J.: Further Studies on a Collagenase in Middle Ear Cholesteatomy. *Ann. Otol.*, 80:177–185, 1971.
3. Allam, A. F.: Pneumatization of the Temporal Bone. *Ann. Otol. Rhinol. Laryngol.*, 78:49–64, 1969.
4. Bartels, L. F. and Sheehy, J. L.: Total Obliteration of the Mastoid, Middle Ear, and External Auditory Canal. A Review of 27 Cases. *Laryngoscope*, 91:1100–1108 (July), 1981.
5. Gacek, R. R.: Mastoid and Middle Ear Cavity Obliteration For Control of Otitis Media. *Ann. Otol. Rhinol. Laryngol.*, 85:309, 1976.
6. Kinney, S. E.: Defensive Chronic Ear Surgery. *Laryngoscope*, 90:1082–1088, 1980.
7. Lee, K. J., and Schuknecht, H. F.: Results of Tympanoplasty and Mastoidectomy at the Massachusetts Eye and Ear Infirmary. *Laryngoscope*, 81:529–543, 1971.
8. Milstein, S.: The History of Mastoid Surgery. *Am. J. Otol.*, 1(3):174–178, 1980.
9. Palva, T.: Mastoid Obliteration. *Acta Otolaryngol. Suppl.*, 360:152–154, 1979.
10. Palva, T. and Virtanen, H.: Ear Surgery and the Mastoid Air Cell System. *Arch. Otolaryngol.* 107:71–73, 1981.
11. Paparella, M. M. and Meyerhoff, W. L.: Mastoidectomy and Tympanoplasty in Otolaryngology, Vol. II, the Ear, M. D. Paparella and D. A. Shumrick (Eds.). Saunders, Philadelphia, 1980.
12. Shambaugh, G. E., Jr., and Glasscock, M. E., III.: Surgery of the Ear, 3rd ed. Saunders, Philadelphia, 1980.
13. Sheehy, J. L.: Surgery of Chronic Otitis Media in Otolaryngology. Vol. I, G. M. English (Ed.). Harper & Row, New York, 1981.
14. Sheehy, J. L.: Cholesteatoma Surgery in Children. *Acta Oto. Rhino. Laryngologica Belgica*, 34(1), 1980.
15. Sheehy, J. L. and Patterson, M. E.: Intact Canal Wall Tympanoplasty with Mastoidectomy. *Laryngoscope*, 77:1502–1542, 1967.
16. Sheehy, J. L.: The Intact Canal Wall Technique in Management of Aural Cholesteatoma. *J. Laryngol. Otol.*, 84:1–31, 1970.
17. Smith, J. B., and Sullivan, J. A.: The Modified Radical Mastoidectomy. *J. Otolaryngol.*, 9(2):149–154, 1980.

11

Simple Mastoidectomy

K. J. Lee

The postauricular area shown in Figure 11-1 is infiltrated with 1% lidocaine (Xylocaine) with epinephrine 1:100,000 concentration.

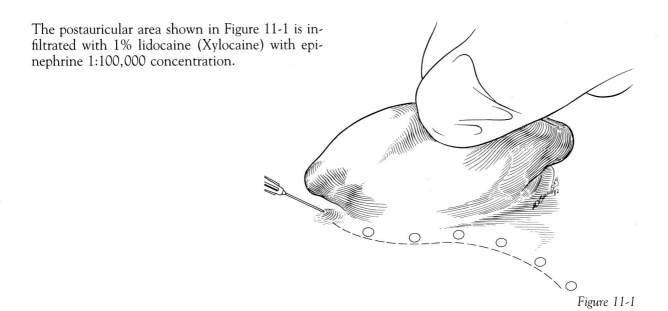

Figure 11-1

205

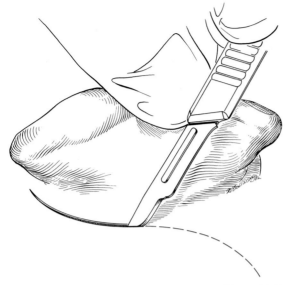

Figure 11-2

In performing a simple mastoidectomy in an infant, it is necessary to place the postauricular incision more posteriorly in the inferior aspect to avoid damaging the facial nerve (Figure 11-2). The mastoid process and tympanic ring are not fully developed and ossified. In older children and in adults, an incision is made 0.5–1 cm posterior to the crease (see Chapter 12). The posterior bony canal is preserved. A complete simple mastoidectomy is done to evacuate the pus as well as to safely remove as much of the granulation tissue and osteitic bone as possible. The periantral cells, sinodural area, mastoid tip, epitympanum, and tegmen should be methodically inspected and cleaned.

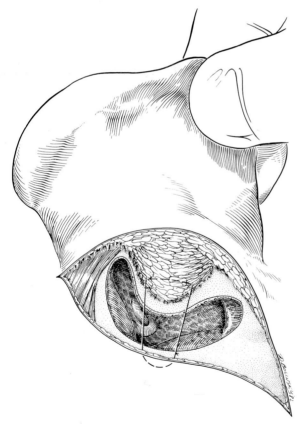

Figure 11-3

A mattress stitch of 3-0 chromic catgut is placed to bring together the posterior canal skin to the posterior auricular muscle and subcutaneous tissue to avoid a postoperative conchal or meatal collapse (Figure 11-3). The use of a Telfa roll in the external auditory canal helps to prevent this problem. (Chapter 12)

The incision is closed with interrupted 5-0 nylon sutures (Figure 11-4).

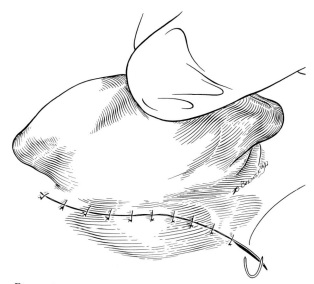

Figure 11-4

12

Mastoidotympanoplasty

K. J. Lee

TECHNIQUE

The postauricular area is infiltrated with 2 ml of 1% lidocaine (Xylocaine) with epinephrine 1:100,000 5–10 minutes before the incision is made (Figure 12-1).

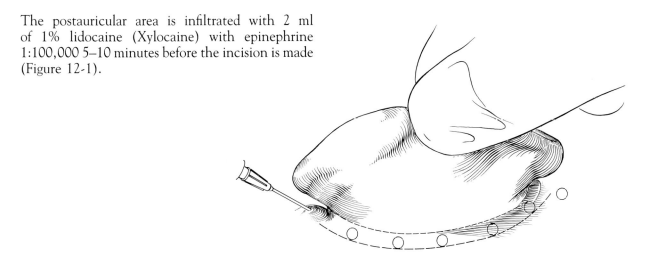

Figure 12-1

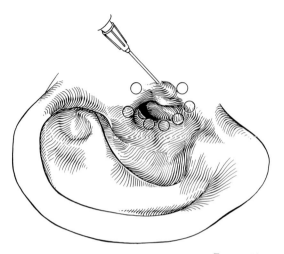

The cartilaginous canal is similarly infiltrated 5–10 minutes before surgery (Figure 12-2). It is also wise to infiltrate the posterior and anterior bony canal walls at this time if the need for an anterior canal skin flap or a tympanomeatal flap is anticipated.

Figure 12-2

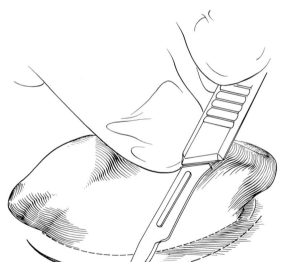

The postauricular incision is made approximately 0.5 cm behind the postauricular crease to avoid the appearance of a plastered auricle postoperatively as well as a depression in the crease (Figure 12-3).

Figure 12-3

After the incision is carried through the full thickness of the skin, dissection of the subcutaneous and
fibrous tissue is performed up to the junction of the
cartilaginous and bony canal with the bovie coagulation cautery set at No. 4 on the Valley Laboratory SSE2-K machine (Figure 12-4). Maximum
hemostasis is achieved if the coagulation setting is
used instead of the cutting setting. In order to make
dissection easier with the coagulation current, it is
essential to retract the auricle anterolaterally, ap-
plying the principle of traction and countertraction.

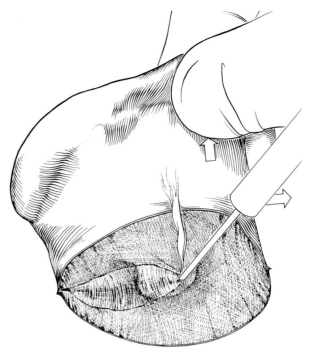

Figure 12-4

A 6–12 o'clock incision is made along the posterior
bony canal, 3–5 mm lateral to the fibrous annulus.
Either a round knife or a lancet knife can be used
for this step of the procedure (Figure 12-5).

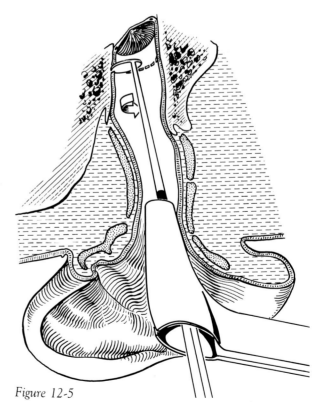

Figure 12-5

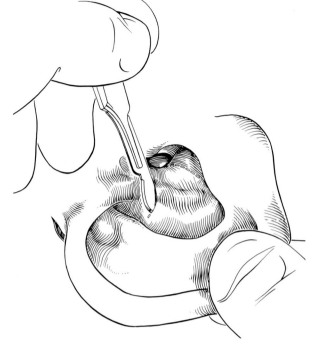

In developing the Körner flap (a posterior full-thickness skin flap based laterally at the concha), an incision is carried from the incision shown in Figure 12-5 to the helical crus (without cutting into it), staying as close to the 12 o'clock position as possible to obtain a broad pedicle flap (Figure 12-6). In view of the thickness of the soft tissue and the cartilage encountered, it is wise to use a fresh sharp blade and cut in a gentle see-saw motion. A firm push to cut through this dense tissue may accidentally transect the auricle, an unnecessary complication. A similar incision is made inferiorly at the 6 o'clock position.

This gentle see-saw technique is facilitated by holding the auricle anterolaterally. An extra snip by the curved Stevens scissors at both the superior and inferior attachments to the concha further releases the Körner flap (Figure 12-7).

Figure 12-6

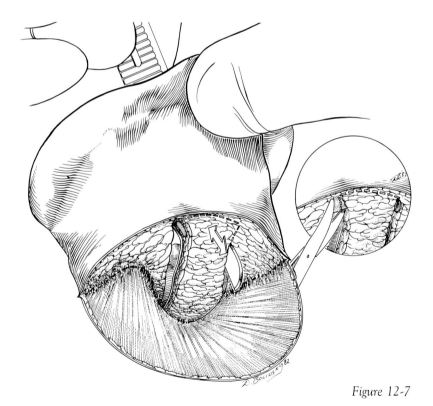

Figure 12-7

The broad-based pedicle flap (Körner) is shown in Figure 12-8. Excess adipose-connective tissue is trimmed off with a No. 11 blade. A mosquito snap offers countertraction. Care should be taken to avoid "buttonholing" the flap.

With the index finger in the external auditory meatus pushing posteriorly, a generous crescent of conchal cartilage is removed with a No. 15 blade to effect a wide meatoplasty (sketch in Figure 12-9A; photograph in Figure 12-9B). It is again important not to buttonhole the pedicle.

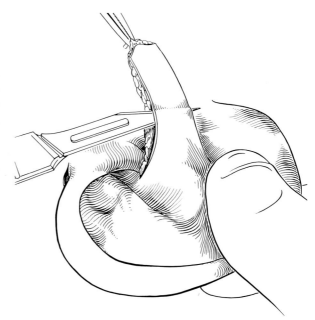

Figure 12-8

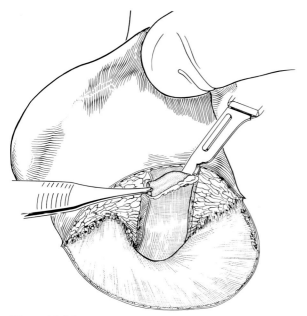

Figure 12-9A

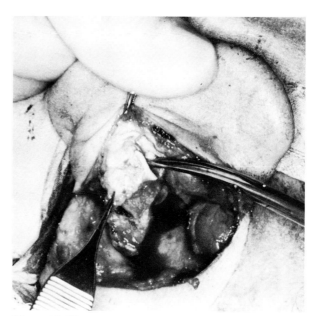

Figure 12-9B

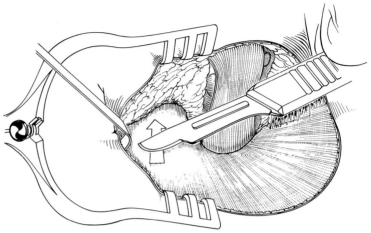

Figure 12-10

A self-retaining retractor is placed as shown in Figure 12-10, and with the help of a rack retractor, the temporalis muscle with its fascia is exposed. With a sweeping motion, areolar tissues are removed and discarded, exposing the white glistening temporalis fascia. (Suffice it to mention that there are otologists who use the prefascia tissue for tympanoplasty graft.)

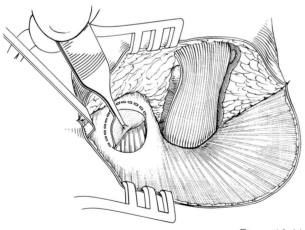

As shown in Figure 12-11, an oval-shaped incision is made just through the fascia. By use of a small, flat periosteal elevator, the muscle fibers and any vessels are swept away from the undersurface of the fascia to obtain a fascia graft unencumbered by extraneous tissues. This maneuver further prevents bleeding by separating the vessels atraumatically from the undersurface of the fascia.

Figure 12-11

If the graft obtained is too thick, a No. 15 blade is used to remove the excess subcutaneous, adipose, or muscular tissues in a scraping fashion (Figure 12-12). A 4 × 4 gauze gives firm countertraction. Keep the graft moist. (Some surgeons prefer a "parchment dry" graft.)

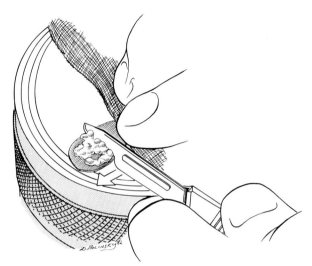

Figure 12-12

The inferiorly based muscle pedicle flap is made with the coagulation current set at No. 4 on the Valley Laboratory SSE2-K machine (Figure 12-13).

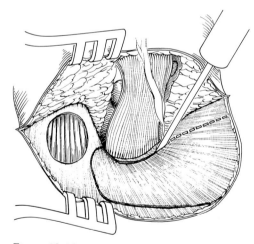

Figure 12-13

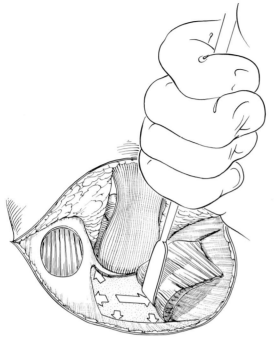

With the use of a Lempert elevator, the inferiorly based muscle pedicle flap is elevated (Figure 12-14).

It is important to elevate sufficiently in the anterior and superior directions (Figure 12-15). One of the common errors is "searching" for the antrum too inferiorly or too posteroinferiorly, causing damage to the horizontal semicircular canal or to the facial nerve.

Figure 12-14

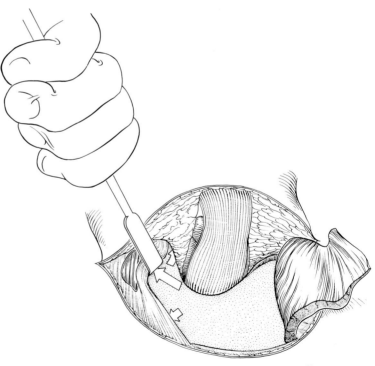

Figure 12-15

With the Lee-Stryker drill (or any other similar drill), the mastoid cortex is removed. Given any drill system, the straight handpiece usually rotates at a higher rpm and thus is preferred for initial drilling of the harder mastoid bone. Using an angle drill with a lower rpm may diminish the life span of the handpiece. A 20° angled handpiece should be used later for the more delicate drilling and when better visualization is necessary (Figure 12-16).

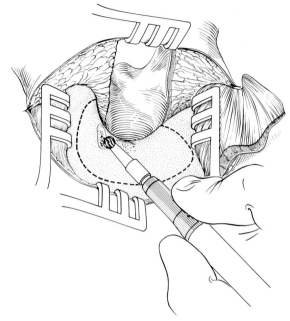

Figure 12-16

The direction of the drilling is as shown by the arrows in Figure 12-17. Care should be taken to adequately expose the sinodural angle, the epitympanum, the "zygomatic root" region, and the mastoid tip. It is desirable to get close to the tegmen without exposing the dura. Properly identifying the superior margin of dissection avoids entering the antrum in the vicinity of the inferior portion of the horizontal semicircular canal. Missing the antrum and continuing to search for it may damage the horizontal semicircular canal or the facial nerve.

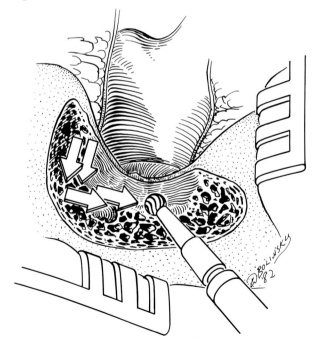

Figure 12-17

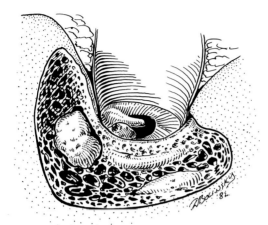

The cholesteatoma is seen through the periantrum cells in Figure 12-18. The sigmoid sinus is exposed. The posterior bony canal has been removed partially.

Figure 12-18

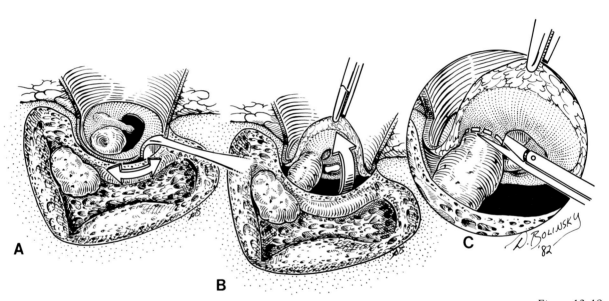

Figure 12-19

In Figure 12-19A the cholesteatoma is visualized through the posterior-superior perforation of the tympanic membrane as well. A tympanomeatal flap is raised with a round knife or lancet knife. In Figure 12-19B the tympanomeatal flap is displaced anteriorly, exposing the cholesteatoma. As shown in Figure 12-19C, the cholesteatoma sac is carefully separated from "normal" tissues with Bellucci scissors.

When removing cholesteatoma, the following principles must be adhered to:

1. Remove all cholesteatoma and remnants of squamous debris.
2. Do not mobilize the footplate.
3. Squamous debris on the footplate can be gently removed with a 0.3-mm hook or a Hough hoe.
4. Check the protympanum, epitympanum, eustachian tube orifice, hypotympanum, facial recess, sinus tympani, sinodural angle, and mastoid tip.
5. In order to adequately visualize the protympanum, elevate the table and rotate the patient away from the surgeon.
6. In order to adequately visualize the posterior aspect of the tympanic cavity, lower the table and rotate the patient toward the surgeon.
7. At times it is necessary to observe the sinus tympani from the head of the table. A small middle ear mirror is helpful.

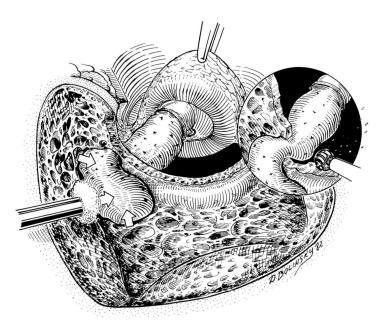

Figure 12-20

Gentle dissection is achieved with a cotton pledget at the tip of a Baron No. 5 suction or held by a cup forcep (Figure 12-20). The facial ridge is lowered to clean the facial recess cells and to better visualize the sinus tympani, two areas in which cholesteatoma is often left unremoved. The bridge is taken down slowly with a diamond burr until a "paper-thin" layer of bone remains. Care is exercised not to touch the incus, which, if still articulating with a normal stapes, may induce a high-frequency sensory neural hearing loss. During the drilling, care should also be exercised to avoid damage to the facial nerve, which may be dehiscent. The paper-thin bridge that is left after the drilling is finally removed with a small periosteal elevator or a Buckingham duckbill.

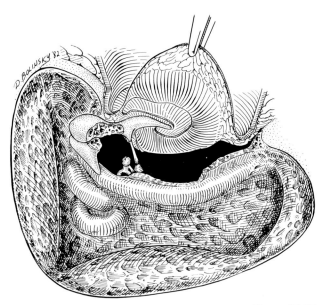

Figure 12-21

The facial nerve and the horizontal and posterior semicircular canals are exposed. The partially necrosed malleus and incus as well as the stapes are seen in Figure 12-21. In exposing the epitympanum and removing the cholesteatoma from the epitympanum, care must be exercised so as not to damage the facial nerve, in the tympanic (horizontal) portion as well as in the vicinity of the geniculate ganglion. Proximal to the tympanic portion of the facial nerve, the nerve lies in the medial wall of the epitympanum. At the conclusion of the mastoidectomy, the anterior and posterior buttresses should be removed. The facial ridge should be lowered. There should be no rough or irregular edges.

The edges of the perforation are freshened with a Rosen needle (Figure 12-22).

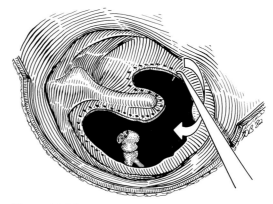

Figure 12-22

The edges are cleaned with cup forceps (Figure 12-23).

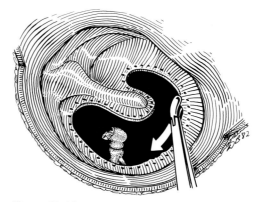

Figure 12-23

The undersurface is scored to remove all squamous epithelium (Figure 12-24).

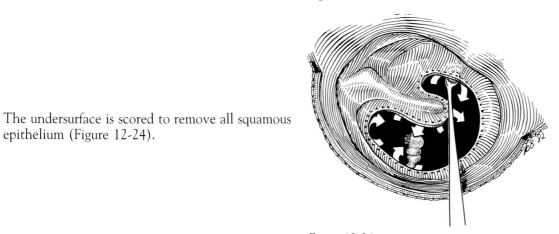

Figure 12-24

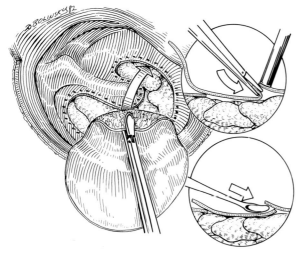

The middle-ear space is packed with Gelfoam pledgets soaked in Cortisporin drops (or left dry, depending on the surgeon's preference (Figure 12-25). The temporalis fascia is grasped with a cup forceps and led to the undersurface of the anterior margin of the perforation. With the help of a small, smooth alligator forceps or a Buckingham duckbill, the graft is led anteriorly carefully. With the help of the Baron No. 3 suction, the drum remnant can be gently lifted to ease the placement of the graft.

Figure 12-25

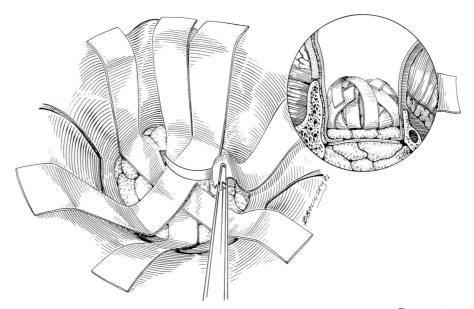

Figure 12-26

Gelfoam pledgets soaked in Cortisporin are placed lateral to the graft and tympanic membrane (Figure 12-26). Strips of Owen's silk soaked in Cortisporin are then folded over the Gelfoam to form a bolus packing.

The inferiorly based muscle pedicle flap is placed in the mastoid cavity to help reduce the cavity size (Figure 12-27). This technique is utilized only if no known cholesteatoma is left behind. In a large cavity, some surgeons add an anterosuperiorly based muscle pedicle flap to reduce the cavity size. However, it is the author's technique to usually obliterate only the inferior aspect of the cavity. Care should always be exercised to remove all cholesteatoma. In most instances, any squamous epithelium left unknowingly is usually in the upper portion of the cavity such as in the vicinity of the sinodural angle and tegmen mastoidii. The inferior aspect of the cavity is also the area subjected to postoperative debris accumulation leading to reinfection. Hence it is wise to reduce the cavity size by obliterating the cavity with an inferiorly based pedicle flap. Careful reduction of cavity size by obliterating the spaces free of disease is not to be confused with "blindly" obliterating the whole cavity and middle ear and hence introducing the possibility of burying disease.

The muscle pedicle flaps become a fibrotic mass, reducing the cavity size. It can never completely obliterate the mastoid cavity. Together with a wide meatoplasty, the surgeon is merely converting a "narrow-mouthed" opening leading to a large empty space into a "wide-mouthed" opening leading to a space of approximately the same diameter. The Körner flap supplies the pedicle skin for early epithelization and healing.

The incision is then closed without a drain (Figure 12-28).

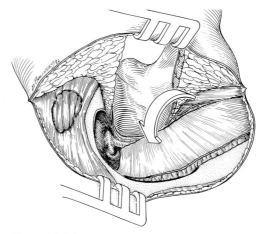

Figure 12-27

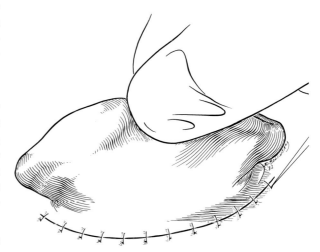

Figure 12-28

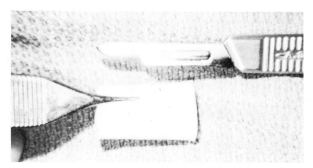

Figure 12-29

A Telfa roll is made as shown in Figure 12-29.

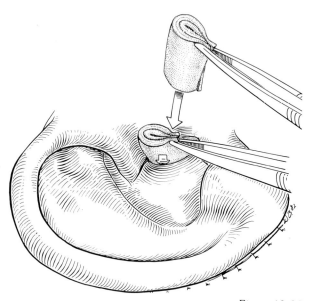

Figure 12-30

This Telfa roll is carefully tucked into the external auditory canal to serve as an outer packing (Figure 12-30). Care should be taken not to curl the Körner flap.

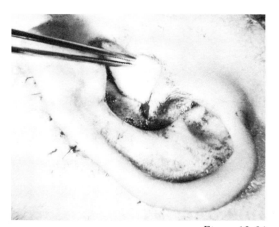

Figure 12-31

Subsequently, a tight mastoid dressing is placed (Figure 12-31). This is removed in 48 hours and replaced with cotton balls and bandaids.

The Telfa roll and the postauricular stitches are removed in 1 week, while the Owen's silk is removed in 2 weeks. Any granulation tissue is cauterized with silver nitrate and painted with gentian violet. The patient is seen once a week for a while to ascertain proper epithelization to achieve a safe, dry ear. Repeated cauterization and application of gentian violet may be necessary.

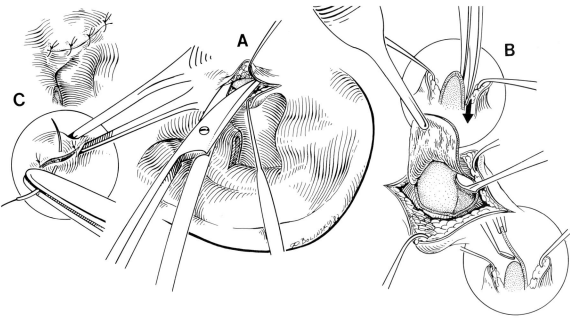

Figure 12-32

ALTERNATIVE PROCEDURES

Instead of temporalis fascia, tragal perichondrium can be used for tympanoplasty. After infiltration with 1% Xylocaine with epinephrine 1:100,000, the skin incision is made, and the tragal cartilage with its perichondrium is freed (Figure 12-32A). With a round knife or lancet knife, the cartilage together with the perichondrium is exposed (Figure 12-32B). Subsequently, the perichondrium is dissected free as one large piece of perichondrium. The incision is closed with 5-0 nylon sutures (Figure 12-32C).

A graft can be placed laterally as shown in Figure 12-33. When placing the graft laterally, it is of utmost importance that the epithelium is completely removed from the lateral surface of the tympanic membrane.

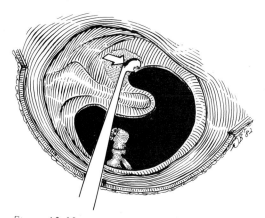

Figure 12-33

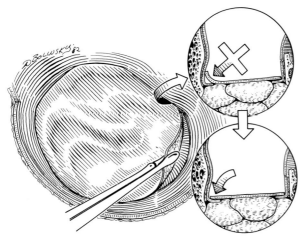

Figure 12-34

The graft should be placed up to the anterior canal wall but should not be permitted to ascend the anterior canal wall, as this may lead to anterior blunting (Figure 12-34). Further lateral migration may lead to lateral graft displacement causing poor ossicular contact.

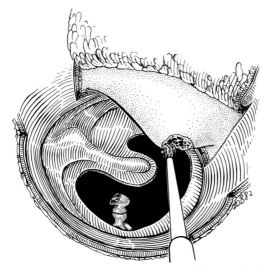

Figure 12-35

Whenever there is an anterior bony canal bulge, it is wise to raise a laterally based anterior canal skin flap and remove the bony bulge with the 20° or 30° angled Lee-Stryker drill (or any similar drill) (Figure 12-35).

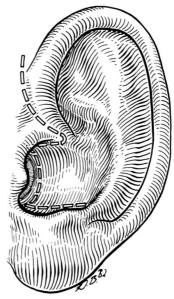

An endaural incision for mastoidotympanoplasty is illustrated in Figure 12-36. In inexperienced hands, this approch does not provide a wide field approach as advocated by Lee and Schuknecht.[1]

Figure 12-36

DISCUSSION

Regarding the step illustrated in Figure 12-35, another technique for preventing anterior blunting or lateral displacement of the graft is to place the graft medial to the anterior fibrous annulus. This is not always technically feasible.

The author prefers a medially placed graft except in cases when there is only a minimal or no anterior tympanic membrane remnant. In such a condition, a medially placed graft may displace itself into the protympanum or eustachian tube orifice leading to a perforation. Hence, the author uses a laterally placed graft in such an instance, care being taken in both the placement of the graft and the packing to avoid anterior blunting or laterally displaced graft.

Generally, the use of Telfa roll for outer packing is preferred to using Nu-gauze strips or vaseline gauze. It can be removed painlessly and without causing any bleeding. It also produces minimal granulation tissues.

REFERENCES

1. Lee, K. J. and Schuknecht, H. F.: Results of Tympanoplasty and Mastoidectomy at the Massachusetts Eye and Ear Infirmary. *Laryngoscope*, 81:529–543, 1971.
2. Schuknecht, H. F., Chasin, W. D., and Kurkjian, J. M.: Stereoscopic Atlas of Mastoidotympanoplastic Surgery, Mosby, St. Louis, 1966.

13

Radical and Modified Radical Mastoidectomy

Eiji Yanagisawa
Myles L. Pensak

INDICATIONS IN 1982

As a result of advanced antibiotic therapy, indications for radical mastoidectomy have diminished during the past decades. Today many otologists feel that even for those patients with a large tympanic membrane perforation with ossicular destruction and cholesteatoma, classic radical mastoidectomy should not be performed when cochlear reserve is good as determined by accurate audiometric testing. The eustachian tube should not be closed, tympanic mucosa should not be curetted, nor should ossicular and tympanic membrane remnants be removed, as required in classic radical mastoidectomy, for these will be needed for future tympanoplasty.

The following are considered to be indications for radical mastoidectomy today: (1) chronic otorrhea due to secondary acquired cholesteatoma with profound sensorineural hearing loss; (2) chronic otorrhea due to chronic perilabyrinthine osteitis with a scant foul discharge and chronic pain deep in the ear, in which the tympanum, hypotympanum, and peritubal area, in addition to the mastoid, attic, and perilabyrinthine areas, need to be explored; and (3) carcinoma of the external meatus and middle ear, which requires a radical mastoidectomy with removal of most of the temporal bone while preservation of hearing is of secondary importance.

Radical mastoidectomy is also indicated for the immune compromised patient with uncontrolled middle-ear and mastoid infections in whom persistent infection or multiple staged operations may carry a high morbidity or mortality rate.

The Bondy type of modified radical mastoidectomy is indicated for cholesteatoma with chronic aural drainage in which cochlear reserve is sufficient for contemplation of future tympanoplasty and where exteriorization of the cholesteatoma is desired. Modified radical mastoidectomy is the basic procedure of choice by the authors for surgery for chronic otitis media with attic or antral cholesteatoma. It should be emphasized that effective tympanoplastic reconstruction with excellent functional results can be achieved with this operation. This procedure is particularly recommended for the occasional surgeon who is not familiar with "canal wall-up" techniques.

SURGICAL TECHNIQUE

RADICAL MASTOIDECTOMY

A standard postauricular incision is made and carried down to the mastoid cortex (Figure 13-1A). Retractors are placed, giving optimal exposure of the cortical region (Figure 13-1B). Temporalis fascia may be harvested at this time for grafting subsequently. Hemostasis is achieved with Bovie electrocoagulation. A T-shaped incision is made on the mucoperiosteum overlying the mastoid cortex (Figure 13-1B). The anterior-posterior limb is cut at the level of the linear temporalis. The superior-inferior limb is directed medial to the skin incision. Periosteum is reflected with a Lempert elevator directed at right angles to the mastoid bone (Figure 13-1C). (Note the exposure of the zygomatic root anteriorly.)

The membranous canal is entered by incising the posterior canal wall (*not* the *anterior* canal wall) at the level of the mastoid cortex from a 12 o'clock to a 6 o'clock position (Figure 13-1D). The posterior canal wall skin flap is outlined (Figure 13-1E). The skin flap is elevated as an inferolaterally based pedicle; this is tacked down with a suture to avoid avulsion (Figure 13-1F).

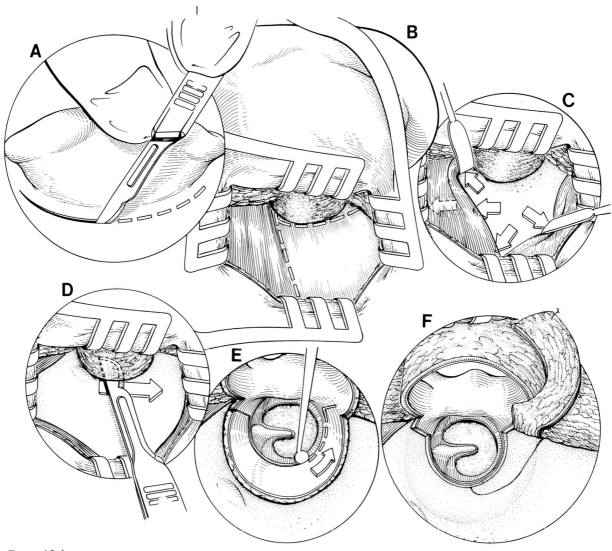

Figure 13-1

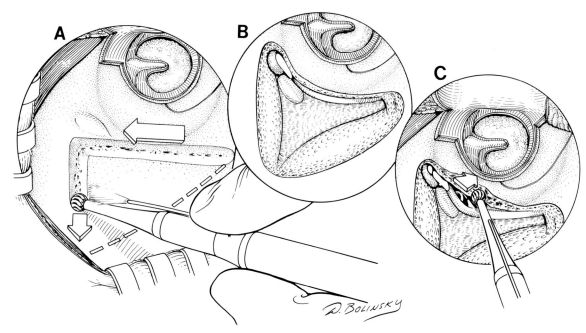

Figure 13-2

A cortical mastoidectomy is performed, using a large cutting burr (Figure 13-2A). The sinodural angle (Citelli's angle) is defined posterior-superiorly. The sigmoid sinus is defined but not "blue-lined." At this point the posterior canal wall is thinned but not reduced. The antrum is opened as shown in Figure 13-2B. Note that the drilling strokes should be done in the direction of the burr spin and parallel to a given anatomic structure at any given point in the mastoid exenteration.

The posterior canal wall is taken down (Figure 13-2C). The ridge of bone should be reduced to the medial extent that defines the bony facial canal. The tympanomeatal flap may be elevated or the tympanic membrane removed.

The "bridge" that overlies the lateral epitympanum is removed with a curette (Figure 13-3). Strokes removing bone should be firm, but controlled and directed laterally away from the dura and facial nerve.

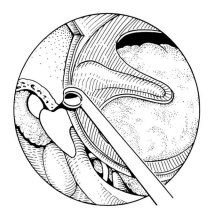

Figure 13-3

The bridge has been removed, and granulation tissue is appreciated in the mesotympanum extending into the epitympanum and antrum (Figure 13-4). The incudostapedial joint is disarticulated, and the incus (or remnant) thereof is removed.

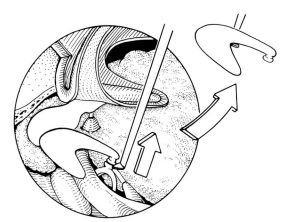

Figure 13-4

The anterior epitympanum is noted and the malleus head is removed using the House-Dieter malleus nipper (Figure 13-5).

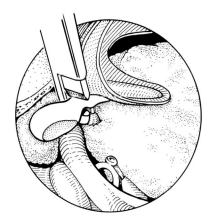

Figure 13-5

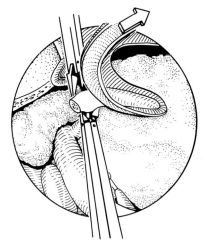

The tensor tympani tendon is cut along with the anterior malleolar ligament (Figure 13-6). The manubrium is removed.

Figure 13-6

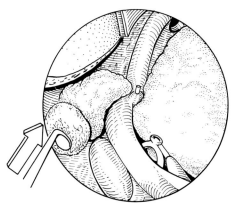
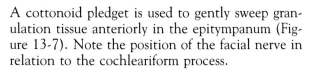

A cottonoid pledget is used to gently sweep granulation tissue anteriorly in the epitympanum (Figure 13-7). Note the position of the facial nerve in relation to the cochleariform process.

Figure 13-7

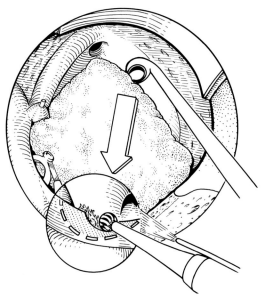

Granulation tissue is evacuated from the middle ear (Figure 13-8). The sinus tympani, lying medial to the facial recess, is a frequent site of retained infected middle-ear mucosa. Often the bone overlying this must be removed. If possible, identification of the pyramidal eminence should be made.

Figure 13-8

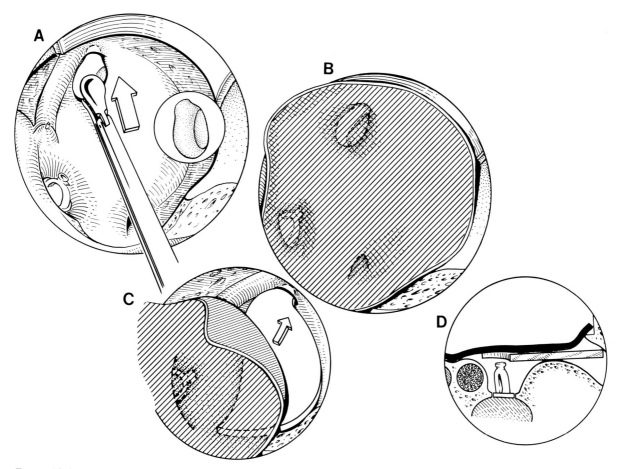

Figure 13-9

Traditionally, following the extirpation of disease from the middle ear, the eustachian tube has been plugged. The malleus head shown in Figure 13-9A is being placed into the anterior mesotympanic entrance of the eustachian tube. A fascia graft is placed over the evacuated middle ear (Figure 13-9B). A thin graft will heal more readily than a thick graft, provided the surgeon does not "cover up" infected mucosa.

As tympanoplastic techniques improve, the hope for middle-ear reconstruction and functional salvage becomes a factor in the surgical technique employed at the time of mastoidectomy. Currently, it is advisable, especially in younger patients, to maintain the patency of the eustachian tube.

Figure 13-9C shows Silastic sheeting being placed from the eustachian tube anteriorly to the round-window niche in the hypotympanum. A fascia graft is placed over this sheeting. Figure 13-9D shows the relative positions of the graft and sheeting.

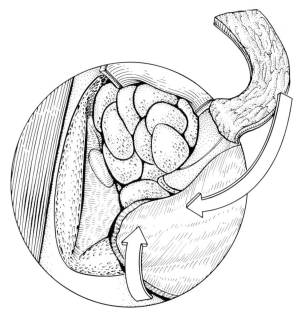

Gelfoam is placed in the cavity medially while a musculoplasty reduces the size of the residual cavity (Figure 13-10). The inferiorly based skin flap is repositioned.

Figure 13-10

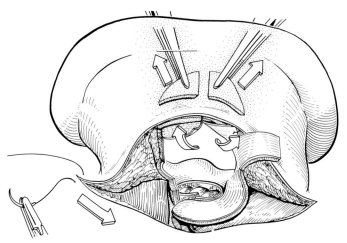

Figure 13-11

A meatoplasty is performed to ensure adequate visualization for the safe and efficient cleansing and inspection of the mastoid bowl (Figure 13-11).

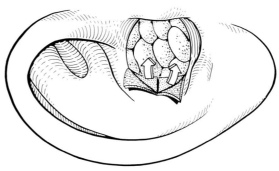

Figure 13-12

As shown in Figure 13-12 and Figure 13-13, the meatal opening is established by removal of wedges of conchal cartilage and attendant soft tissue with preservation of the posterior canal wall skin as described in Figure 13-32.

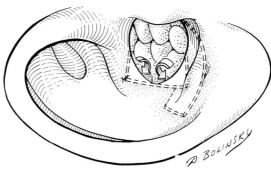

Figure 13-13

MODIFIED RADICAL MASTOIDECTOMY (SHAMBAUGH AND GLASSCOCK)

With a No. 15 blade, a standard Lempert endaural incision is made following local infiltration with anesthetic injection (Figure 13-14). (*Note:* Exposure for the procedure may be gained by Heerman's endaural incision or from a standard postauricular incision.)

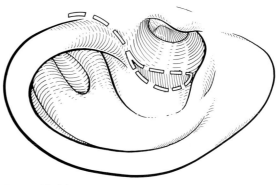

Figure 13-14

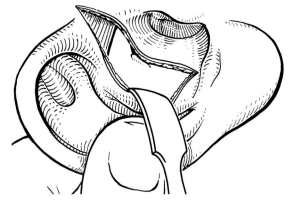

Figure 13-15

With the use of a Lempert periosteal elevator, the root of the zygoma is defined anteriorly as the mastoid cortex is demonstrated posteriorly (Figure 13-15).

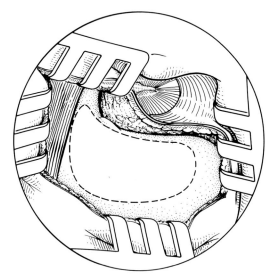

Figure 13-16

Retractors are placed and positioned to afford optimal exposure for the operator (Figure 13-16).

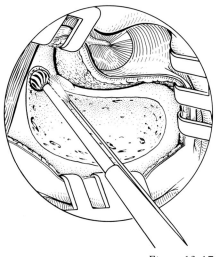

Figure 13-17

By use of a large cutting burr and drilling in the direction of rotation of the burr, the antrum is exposed (Figure 13-17). Broad, smooth strokes are used, and working in a "hole" is to be discouraged. The surgeon should be aware of potential Körner's septum (petrosquamous bony lamina) lying lateral to the antrum. (*Note:* the spine of Henle should direct the surgeon to the antrum.)

The cholesteatoma is seen in Figure 13-18. Subsequently, the sinodural angle is defined and the sigmoid sinus defined. The extent of cavity exposed should be dictated by the size of the cholesteatoma, number of infected cells, and degree of osteitis. (*Note*: the smaller the cavity created, the less work required in postoperative management.) The bridge of bone lateral to the epitympanum should be removed carefully and the position of the facial nerve appreciated.

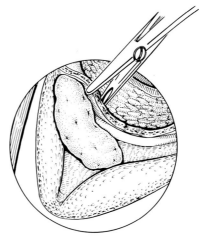

Figure 13-18

Skin of the posterior canal is elevated and reflected antero-inferiorly as a meatal flap is made (Figure 13-19).

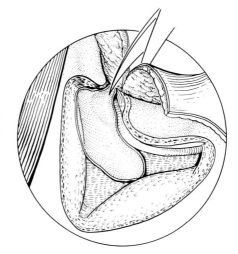

Figure 13-19

Fine curet work or drilling effects dismantling of the remaining bridge of bone posteriorly and inferiorly (bony buttresses) (Figure 13-20). Again note the position of the facial nerve.

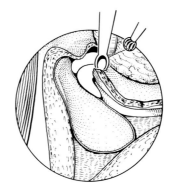

Figure 13-20

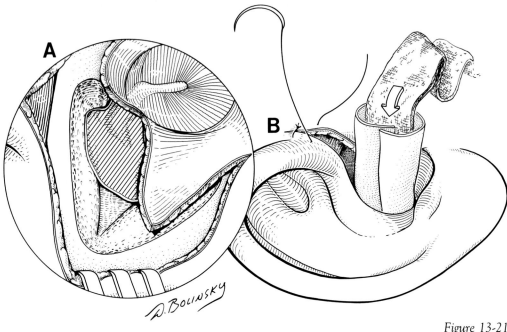

Figure 13-21

The completed cavity is seen in Figure 13-21A. The posterior skin flap is positioned over the facial ridge. Any overlap of flap edge over retained cholesteatoma matrix must be trimmed. When cholesteatoma is completely removed and the ossicular chain is exposed, it should be covered with fascia. Finally, surgical rayon sleeve packing is placed and the endaural incision closed (Figure 13-21B).

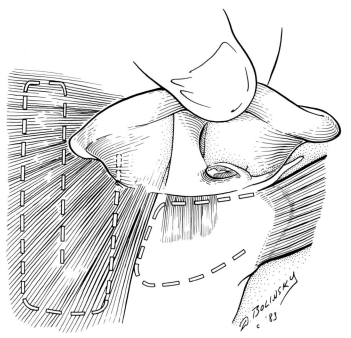

Figure 13-22

MUSCULOPLASTY

The principal objectives are (1) obliteration of the residual cavity, (2) coverage for vital structures (dura superiorly, sigmoid sinus posteriorly, facial ridge medially, horizontal canal medially), (3) maintenance of the cavity and the external auditory canal at the same height for postoperative examination and cleansing, and (4) support of the autograft or homograft posterior canal wall after reconstruction of mastoidectomy cavity.

A superior anteriorly based temporalis muscle flap may be elevated (Figure 13-22). Further muscle may be obtained posteriorly or inferiorly as required.

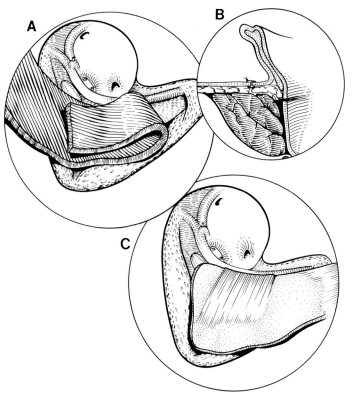

Figure 13-23

The pedicle is swung into the cavity, folded if necessary, and tacked into place. A superiorly based pedicle is shown in Figure 13-23A. Figure 13-23B demonstrates a cross-sectional view of the obliterated mastoid cavity with a musculoplasty. Figure 13-23C shows a muscle-fascia inferiorly based pedicle being positioned.

MEATOPLASTY COMBINED WITH MASTOID SURGERY

KÖRNER'S TECHNIQUE

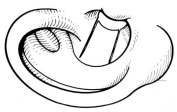

Figure 13-24

A wide posteriorly based canal (cartilaginous) skin flap is elevated (Figure 13-24).

The auricle is reflected anteriorly and the pedicle delivered into the mastoid operative site (Figure 13-25).

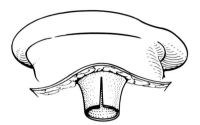

Figure 13-25

Conchal cartilage and attendant soft tissue are removed (Figure 13-26).

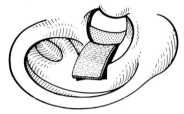

Figure 13-26

The flap is returned to its anatomic position, having been thinned out permitting a wider meatal opening (Figure 13-27).

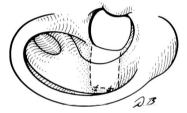

Figure 13-27

FISCH'S TECHNIQUE

A linear incision is carried along the posterior wall (Figure 13-28).

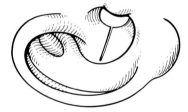

Figure 13-28

The two leaves of the flap are delivered into the postauricular field (Figure 13-29).

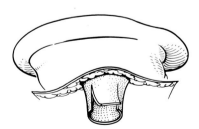

Figure 13-29

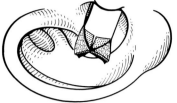

Figure 13-30

Cartilage and soft tissue are removed (Figure 13-30).

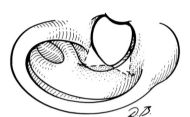

Figure 13-31

The two leaves of the flap, having been thinned, are returned to their anatomic positions (Figure 13-31).

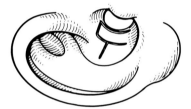

Figure 13-32

YANAGISAWA'S TECHNIQUE

An inferiorly based rectangular flap is created perpendicular to the long axis of the canal in the conchal cartilage and overlying skin. A linear incision is made parallel to this and extended posteriorly (Figure 13-32).

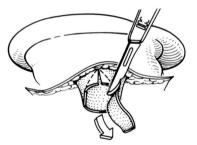

Figure 13-33

The auricle is reflected anteriorly and trilobed flap reflected into the postauricular operative site (Figure 13-33).

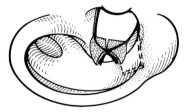

Figure 13-34

Cartilage and soft tissue are skeletonized from the skin flaps (two leaves from the linear incision and one flap from the rectangular design) (Figure 13-34).

The skin is returned to the meatus with the rectangular flap being reflected inferiorly, thus opening the meatus more than with a conventional bilobed skin flap (Figure 13-35).

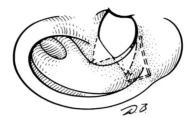

Figure 13-35

SIEBERMAN'S TECHNIQUE

An inverted Y-shaped incision is made in the posterior skin and conchal cartilage (Figure 13-36).

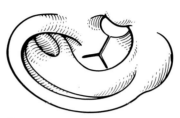

Figure 13-36

The flaps are inverted and pulled into the postauricular operative site (Figure 13-37).

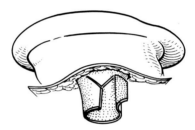

Figure 13-37

Conchal cartilage and soft tissue are removed (Figure 13-38).

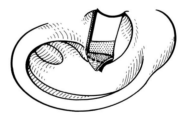

Figure 13-38

The skin is placed down with three corner sutures as the posterior skin flaps over the meatus are placed (Figure 13-39).

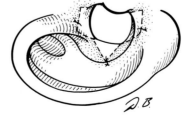

Figure 13-39

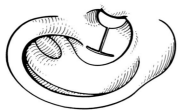

Figure 13-40

PANSE AND PORTMANN'S TECHNIQUE

An inverted T is made in the posterior skin overlying the conchal cartilage (Figure 13-40).

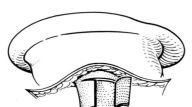

Figure 13-41

The flaps are reflected into the postauricular operative site (Figure 13-41).

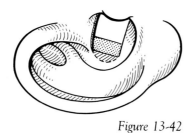

Figure 13-42

Conchal cartilage and soft tissue are removed (Figure 13-42).

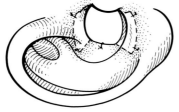

Figure 13-43

At the time of skin replacement, the T is opened up and sutured into the new meatus with four quadrant sutures (Figure 13-43).

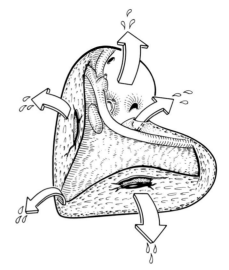

Figure 13-44A

PROBLEMS AND SOLUTIONS

BLEEDING

Bleeding may be encountered in several critical locations within the operative field, including the dura (superior locale), the sinodural angle, the sigmoid sinus, the middle ear, and the facial nerve (Figure 13-44A). Bleeding may be the first indication to the surgeon that dura lies just below his drill (Figure 13-44B). Concomitant to an increase in bleeding, a change in sound or feel of the drill may herald the presence of dura. For bleeding in the sinodural angle, bone wax may be applied quite readily because of the anatomic configuration (Figure 13-44C).

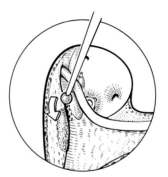

Figure 13-44B

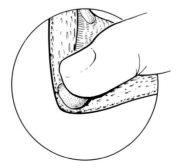

Figure 13-44C

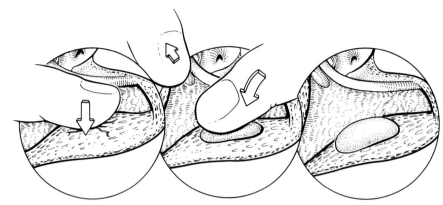

Figure 13-44D

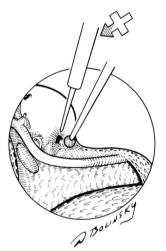

Figure 13-44E

Likewise, exposed bleeding dura may be covered if localized. Larger defects may, once controlled, be covered with autogenous material. Entry into the sigmoid sinus may produce profuse bleeding (Figure 13-44D). Immediate coverage with the index finger will quiet down both the surgeon and the operative field. Bone wax is applied and the procedure continued. At the close of the procedure, the bone wax is removed and a fascia graft covering is placed. (*Note*: While performing a mastoidectomy, the sigmoid sinus may lie anteriorly. Use of a 30-gauge needle will help distinguish the sinus from a questionable air cell.)

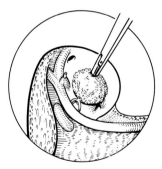

Figure 13-44F

Bleeding around the facial nerve may be controlled with a diamond burr if a bony covering is present (Figure 13-44E). The drill should move only *parallel* to the course of the nerve. Bovie cautery is to be avoided. Bleeding in the middle ear may be controlled with a cotton ball pleget impregnated with adrenalin (1:1000 to 1:100,000) lidocaine (Xylocaine) dilution (Figure 13-44F).

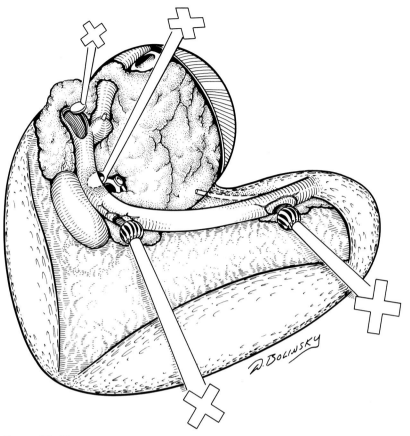

Figure 13-45

FACIAL NERVE INJURY

Injury to the facial nerve can be catastrophic to both patient and surgeon. The potential for injury exists in all mastoidectomy procedures. Risk of injury, however, may be mitigated by following the time-honored axiom that the safest way of avoiding injury to the nerve is by identifying the nerve itself. This concept is amplified in both chronic ear procedures or revision procedures.

As shown in Figure 13-45, four common sites of injury are demonstrated: (1) internal (first) genu and the geniculate ganglion; (2) horizontal segment in the middle ear, where partial dehiscence may occur quite frequently (approximately 50%); (3) at the second genu as the nerve begins its vertical course; and (4) inferiorly, near the stylomastoid foramen.

Injury to the nerve may be avoided by identifying the:

- Geniculate ganglion.
- Cochleariform process and the tensor tympani tendon. The semicanal extends anteriorly while the nerve goes superiorly (forming a V).
- Stapes, oval-window niche, or round-window niche.
- Horizontal semicircular canal.
- Digastric ridge.
- Pyramidal eminence.
- Stylomastoid foramen.

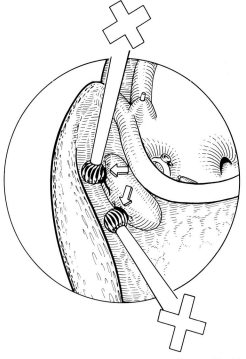

LABYRINTHINE INJURY

Injury to the lateral canal may occur while the surgeon is defining the dura and not being cautious that a burr that is too large may be insulting the labyrinth inferiorly (Figure 13-46).

Figure 13-46

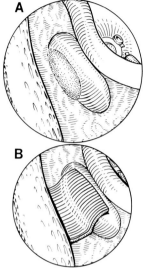

Bone dust is placed over an exposed bony labyrinth (Figure 13-47A). Fascia is placed as an autogenous covering (Figure 13-47B).

Figure 13-47

MUCOUS OR CHOCOLATE CYST

A mucous cyst may present in any portion of the cavity; however, when it lies high in the bowl or along the superior wall of the external canal, one must consider brain herniation in the differential.

The cyst is first evacuated of old blood and mucoid material (Figure 13-48).

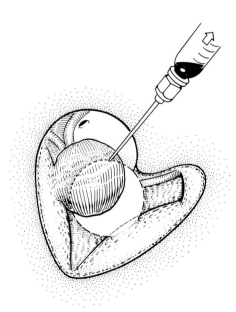

Figure 13-48

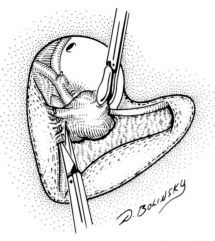

Figure 13-49

Bellucci scissors are then used to excise the cyst (Figure 13-49).

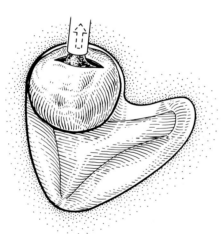

Figure 13-50

CHOLESTEATOMA

Cholesteatoma (recurrent or residual) is perhaps the most common of complications. In Figure 13-50 the sac is incised and its contents evacuated.

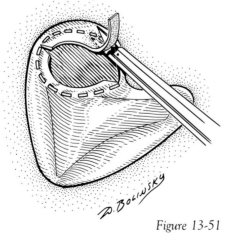

Figure 13-51

The margins of the recurrent sac are sharply cut away, as shown in Figure 13-51. In general this may be performed as an office procedure.

PERSISTENT OTORRHEA

Persistent drainage following mastoid surgery is both upsetting to the patient and frustrating to the surgeon.

Defect in the drum remnant with discharging middle-ear tissue is noted (Figure 13-52).

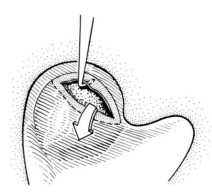

Figure 13-52

The weeping middle-ear tissue is removed and a temporalis fascia graft placed in the medial position (Figure 13-53A). Note the position of the fascia graft shown in Figure 13-53B. Optimally, epithelium will grow over the eustachian tube orifice and seal it, thus eliminating a major source of recurrent drainage (after Brandow[1]).

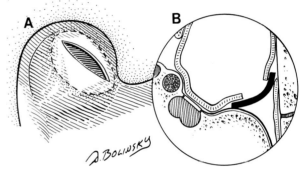

Figure 13-53

STENOSIS OF MASTOID CAVITY

On reexploration years after a proper mastoidectomy had been performed, many experienced otologists have encountered new bone growth, sometimes obliterating the cavity (Figure 13-54).

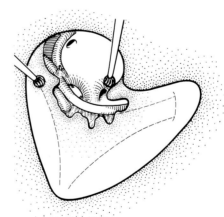

Figure 13-54

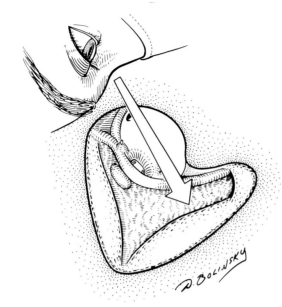

Figure 13-55

The cavity is redefined and the bowl obliterated if need be to establish at one level the external auditory canal and the cavity (Figure 13-55). Only when this is accomplished will prompt, easy care be rendered in postsurgical visits to the office.

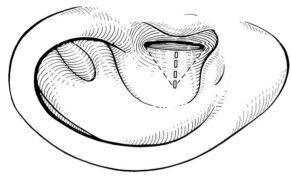

Figure 13-56

MEATAL STENOSIS AND CLOSURE

Stenosis

Narrowing of the ear canal is more commonly seen with the Lempert endaural incision than with the postauricular incision. As scar contraction occurs, the well-defined margins of the external auditory canal narrow (Figure 13-56).

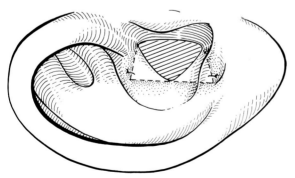

Figure 13-57

By use of a No. 15 Bard-Parker blade or No. 67 Beaver blade, a perpendicular incision is made and conchal cartilage wedges are removed. The skin is tacked down as shown in Figure 13-57.

In some cases almost complete stenosis occurs. In Figure 13-58 an elliptical incision is made along with a perpendicular limb.

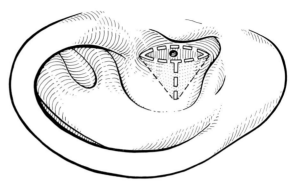

Figure 13-58

In Figure 13-59 cartilage is removed and the skin tacked down posteriorly. Often a small split-thickness skin graft is needed to cover anteriorly.

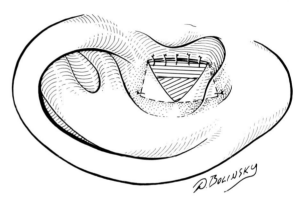

Figure 13-59

Closure

Subtotal meatal closure is noted following an endaural mastoidectomy. An incision is outlined and meatal soft-tissue mass excised (Figure 13-60).

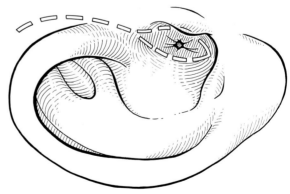

Figure 13-60

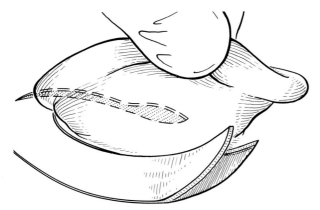

A superiorly based flap is elevated behind the ear, including the dermis and subdermal tissue to afford a better blood supply (Figure 13-61).

Figure 13-61

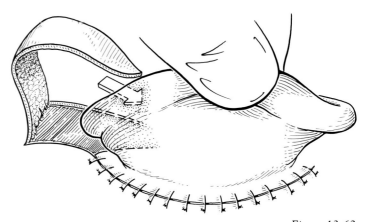

Figure 13-62

The flap is turned into the limb of the No. 3 incision and laid down on the superior bony wall. The postauricular incision is closed primarily (Figure 13-62).

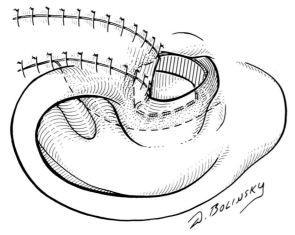

The flap is then sutured into position (Figure 13-63).

Figure 13-63

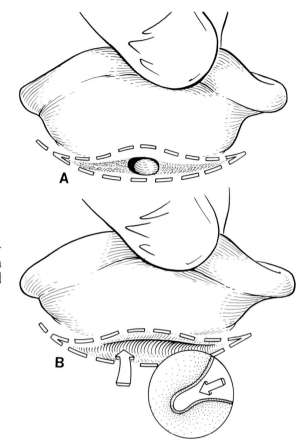

POSTAURICULAR DEPRESSION AND MASTOID CUTANEOUS FISTULA

Two potential long-term complications of the postauricular incision are a mastoid-cutaneous fistula (Figure 13-64A) and retraction into the mastoid cavity of the postauricular skin (Figure 13-64B).

Figure 13-64

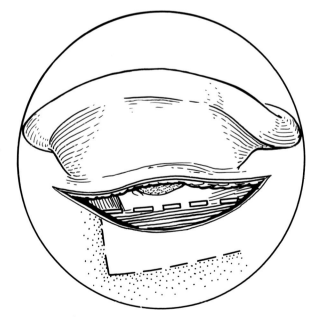

The ear and postauricular region are prepped and draped and the local anesthetic applied. The retracted scar (full thickness) that lies in the depression is excised in an ellipse (Figure 13-65).

Figure 13-65

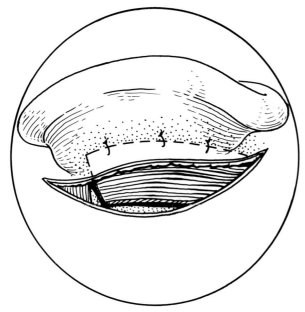

The postauricular skin is undermined, and the auricular skin on the anterior edge of the ellipse is elevated and carried forward onto the chonchal cartilage (Figure 13-66).

Figure 13-66

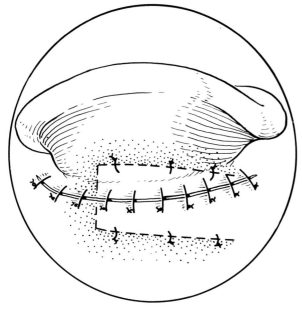

Subcutaneous tissue is advanced in a posterior-to-anterior fashion (Figure 13-67). The flap is freed up with sharp dissection and a needle cautery is used to define its borders. The pedicle remains inferiorly based. Chromic or Dexon sutures fix the advancement flap in place. The skin is closed with nylon sutures.

Figure 13-67

REFERENCES

1. Brandow, E. C., Jr.: Revision surgery for the mastoid cavity. *Otolaryngol. Clin. N. Am.*, 7:41–56, 1974.
2. Kerrison, P.: Diseases of the Ear, 2nd ed. Lippincott, Philadelphia, 1921.
3. Portmann, G.: A Treatise on the Surgical Technique of Otorhinolaryngology, Pierre Viole, (Transl.). William Wood, Baltimore, 1939.
4. Saunders, W. H. and Paparella, M. M.: Atlas of Ear Surgery, 2nd ed., Mosby, St. Louis, 1971.
5. Shambaugh, G. E., Jr. and Glasscock, M. E. III.: Surgery of the Ear, 3rd ed., Saunders, Philadelphia, 1980.

14

Surgery for
————Congenital Anomalies of the Ear————

Eiji Yanagisawa
Myles L. Pensak

Among the many challenges encountered by the otologist, perhaps none presents more philosophical or technical juggernauts than does the patient with congenital anomalies of the ear.

SELECTION OF SURGICAL CANDIDATES

There is probably no one aspect of *congenital aural atresia* that has polarized otologic surgeons more than the controversy over the need for surgery in bilateral atresia only versus unilateral atresia.

We feel that the child with bilateral atresia who by radiographic and audiologic perspective is a surgical candidate should be proposed for surgery be-

tween ages 4 and 6 years. Of paramount importance is the fitting with body-type hearing aids as early as possible along with intense environmental stimulation and language training. Patients with a unilateral deficit should be considered for surgery as teenagers, when they may participate in the decision-making process.

In the case of unilateral pathology, we consider any one or more of the following four factors relative criteria for surgical indication:

1. Tomographic evidence of middle-ear ossicles and a pneumatized mastoid.
2. Recurrent infection.
3. Cholesteatoma.
4. A reasonable degree of certainty that a 30-dB or better air conduction level may be obtained.

261

EMBRYOLOGY

AURICULAR DEVELOPMENT

At the end of the first gestational month, tissue thickening occurs at the dorsal surface of the first branchial groove. This is due to the maturation of the mandibular and hyoid arches.

During weeks 5 and 6, the hillocks (six in number) form from the dorsal tissue thickening observed during week 4. Two hillocks lie anterior to the first groove and four hillocks lie in a posterior position. As the groove develops, the anterior (mandibular arch) hillocks separate from the posterior (hyoid arch) hillocks.

EXTERNAL AUDITORY CANAL AND MIDDLE EAR

The external auditory canal (EAC) is derived from the dorsal aspect of the first groove and lies between the mandibular and hyoid arches. The middle-ear cleft forms from the first pharyngeal pouch along with the auditory tube.

During the seventh week of gestation, the tubotympanic recess from which the middle-ear cleft forms begins to develop laterally from the auditory tube.

The external auditory canal and middle ear are classified according to the following scheme:

- *Group I*: Anomalies are minor. The canal is narrow but patent. The ossicles are fixed and the stapes usually is affected. This type is uncommon, but surgery results are excellent.
- *Group II*: Anomalies are major. The pinna is severely deformed. The external canal is absent, and there are complex middle-ear abnormalities.
- *Group III*: The air-cell system is absent. Cochlear anomalies may be present. Surgery is hazardous, and results are poor.

OSSICLES

The origin of the ossicles are as follows:
- Malleus
  —Head: Arch I
  —Manubrium: Arch II
  —Anterior process: independent ossification center
- Incus
  —Short crus and body: Arch I
  —Long crus: Arch II
- Stapes
  —Head: Arch II
  —Crura: Arch II
  —Bony part of base: Arch II
  —Cartilagenous part of base (otic capsule)

AURAL ATRESIA

CANALPLASTY AND ANTROTOMY

In this approach, the antrum is first entered and well exposed. The horizontal semicircular canal, a most important landmark, and the "ossicular mass" are then identified before removing the atretic plate. The exposure of the antrum will help to prevent the injury to the facial nerve and the ossicles, which may lead to sensorineural deafness.

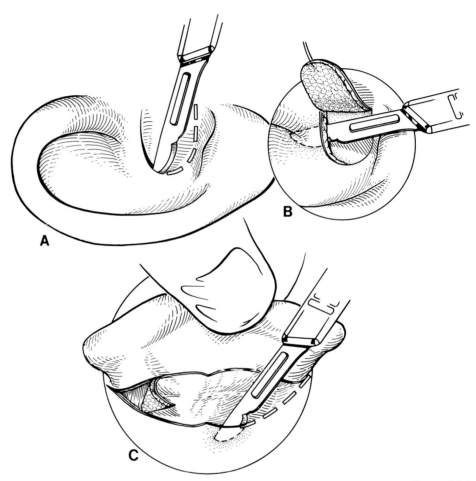

Figure 14-1

A U-shaped skin incision is made anterior to the major portion of the auricle overlying the future site of the lateral portion of the meatus (Figure 14-1A). The incision should be posterior to the superficial temporal artery.

The flap is elevated down to bone and the auricle over the lateral mastoid cortex mobilized (Figure 14-1B).

A postauricular incision is made by excising a wide ellipse of skin. This skin is placed in gauze moistened with physiologic solution and preserved for subsequent use as a free graft (Figure 14-1C).

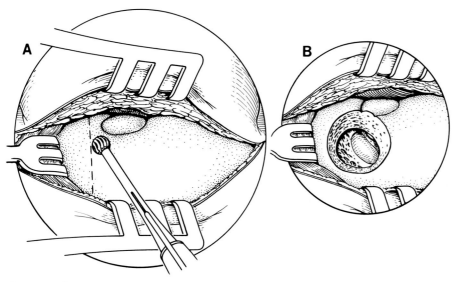

Figure 14-2

The auricle is retracted anteriorly and the lateral mastoid cortex bone exposed (Figure 14-2A). The linea temporalis is defined superiorly, and the root of the zygoma is appreciated anteriorly. Perpendicular to this is the glenoid fossa and mandibular condyle. Often a small bridge of bone may be appreciated lying at this intersection. This bone is the lateral remnant of the tympanic bone. With the dura used as a guide, the antrum is exposed from a superior direction to mitigate the chances of facial nerve injury (Figure 14-2B). The dissection is carried medially and *anteriorly* until the lateral portion of the ossicular mass is appreciated.

The ossicular mass is noted. Inferiorly, the dense bone of the atretic plate must now be cautiously removed to establish a new canal and optimize exposure of the tympanum. A cutting burr is used here (Figure 14-3A) with the operator at all times carefully avoiding direct trauma to the ossicular mass. Figure 14-3B reminds the surgeon to follow the dura medially and anteriorly in the exposure of the antrum.

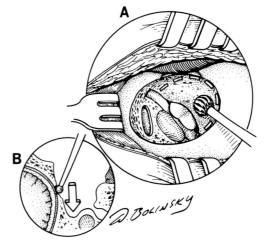

Figure 14-3

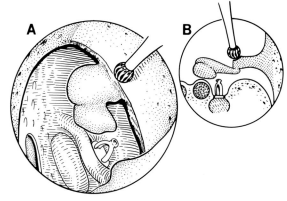

Figure 14-4

The magnified diagram of the removal of the atretic plate lateral to the tympanum shown in Figure 14-4A points out two important features at this juncture: (1) separation of the lateral ossicular mass from the stapes may be present, and recognition of the status of ossicular continuity is of paramount importance; and (2) the atretic plate may be fused to the malleus, and drilling directly on this bony juxtaposition will generate vibratory trauma to the inner ear, if ossicular continuity remains intact (Figure 14-4B).

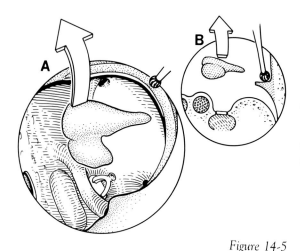

Figure 14-5

The lateral ossicular mass is removed (Figure 14-5A). Figure 14-5B shows a small lip of future anterior canal wall left in place. This will serve as a buttress on which the fascia graft may be laid.

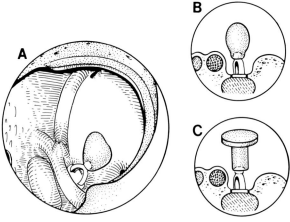

Figure 14-6

Figure 14-6A shows the fully exposed middle ear with smooth margins of the atretic plate defined. Reconstruction (Type III tympanoplasty) may be done with a homograft or autograft ossicle, or by placing a partial ossicular replacement prosthesis (PORP) (Figures 14-6B, C).

A temporalis fascia graft is placed (Figure 14-7).

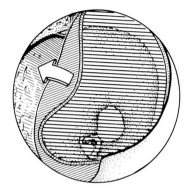

Figure 14-7

The anterior canal flap (see Figure 14-1A) is placed while the harvested skin from the postauricular ellipse is applied as a free split-thickness skin graft to cover the newly created bony canal (Figure 14-8).

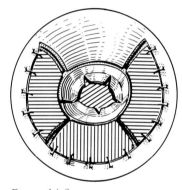

Figure 14-8

Figure 14-9 is a cross-sectional diagram showing ossicular continuity to the membrane graft. Lateral to this the skin grafts have covered the new bony canal. The skin grafts include both the free postauricular graft and split-thickness grafts from the abdomen or arm.

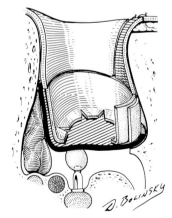

Figure 14-9

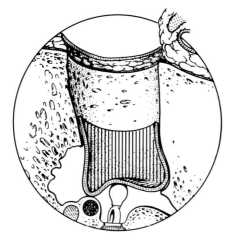

Jahrsdoerfer's Canal Lining Technique

After a middle-ear space with successful ossicular reconstruction has been established, a temporalis fascia graft is placed as shown in Figure 14-10. Note the small bony edges on which the graft is laid within the newly created canal.

Figure 14-10

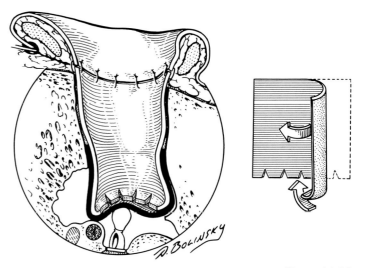

Figure 14-11

The canal is lined by a STSG harvested from the abdominal wall (approximately 6 cm × 6 cm., 0.018 inch thick). The medial border of the skin graft is scalloped to permit easy symmetrical and smooth placement in the canal and in the newly grafted tympanic membrane (Figure 14-11 insert). The goal of the skin graft central fenestration is to allow a thin layer of squamous epithelium to grow over the membrane.

CANALPLASTY

Although this technique may afford the patient the possibility of an optimal closure of the air–bone gap, the procedure is technically difficult. This operation should be undertaken only by the most skilled and experienced otologists since the anatomic landmarks available are limited and direct trauma to the ossicular mass may readily be transmitted to the inner ear. Cosmetically, it is an excellent otologic complementary procedure.

By defining the root of the zygoma, the glenoid fossa anteriorly, and the anterior wall of the mastoid cortex posteriorly, a canal has been extended medially to the tympanum through the atretic plate. A Type III tympanoplasty has been performed in the case shown in Figure 14-12.

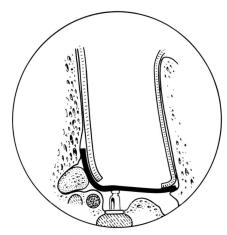

Figure 14-12

In cases such as that shown in Figure 14-13, where the ossicular mass remains intact, the graft should be placed lateral to the ossicular chain.

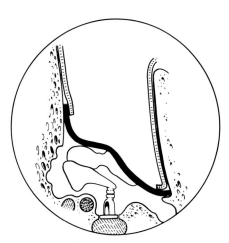

Figure 14-13

MASTOIDECTOMY AND TYMPANOPLASTY

The mastoidectomy-tympanoplasty technique is perhaps the safest procedure in congenital atretic cases. Nevertheless, a high degree of surgical skill is needed to ensure the safe execution of this procedure, and the occasional operator may wish to refer this type of case to a more experienced colleague or ask for assistance.

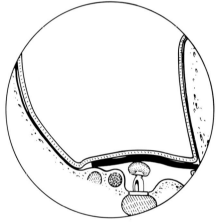

Figure 14-14

In the case shown in Figure 14-14, the mastoid cavity, antrum, and atretic plate have been exposed and opened. There is no need to attempt to define the sinodural angle or sigmoid sinus in these cases (unless infected cells are present). A small cavity will lend itself to easier management. A Type III columella (homograft) strut is shown in Figure 14-14.

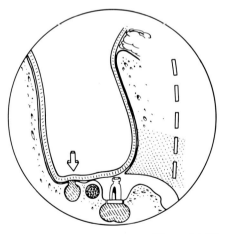

Figure 14-15

A further advantage of the mastoidectomy approach is that in the event that ossicular continuity or oval window grafting is not successful, the surgeon may perform a fenestration of the lateral semicircular canal. In Figure 14-15 note that if a fenestration is preferred as the procedure of choice, there is no need to remove the entire atresia plate.

HOMOGRAFT CANALPLASTY

A canalplasty may be done and ossicular discontinuity noted (Figure 14-16). The ossicular mass may be removed.

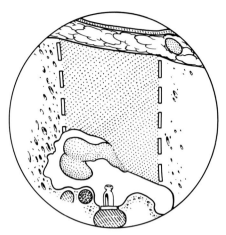

Figure 14-16

A homograft tympanic membrane ossicular chain graft may be used. In Figure 14-17 note positioning of Gelfoam in the newly defined tympanum to support the homograft.

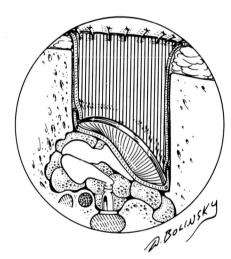

Figure 14-17

MIDDLE-EAR ANOMALIES

Restoration of hearing in the patient with a congenital middle ear anomaly challenges the otologist in both degree of surgical acumen and creative application of tympanoplastic technique. Certain defects may appear "unexplainable" embryologically, especially in view of the "newer theories" of ossicular embryogenesis. Nevertheless, this discussion reflects some of the fundamental surgical tenets and techniques that may be employed when dealing with congenital aberrations.

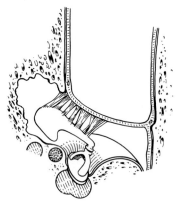

Figure 14-18

MALLEUS ANOMALIES

A young patient with significant A–B gap was explored and found to have an absence of the malleus (Figure 14-18). Fibrous adhesions were attendent to the tympanic membrane and incus.

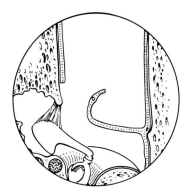

Figure 14-19

The adhesions are cleared from the incus, and as the tympanic membrane is reflected off, care is taken not to introduce squamous epithelium into the middle ear (Figure 14-19).

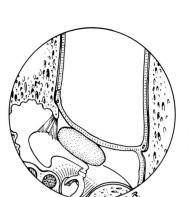

Figure 14-20

A cartilage graft with attendant perichondrium is placed as a strut (Figure 14-20). An excellent result has been obtained.

INCUS ANOMALIES

The long process of the incus may be foreshortened along with a distorted stapes suprastructure (Figure 14-21).

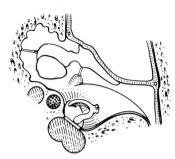

Figure 14-21

Sculptured malleus homograft is employed to bridge the gap from the manubrium to the footplate (Figure 14-22). Note that the stapes suprastructure is left undisturbed.

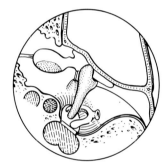

Figure 14-22

An alternative technique (Fisch) places a TORP with cartilage partially against the malleus and partially in contact with the tympanic membrane (Figure 14-23). Medially, the TORP rests on the footplate.

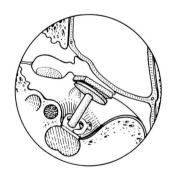

Figure 14-23

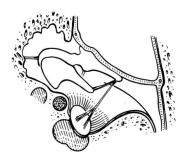

Figure 14-24

STAPES ANOMALIES

Absence of Suprastructure

Illustrating a second arch defect, fibrous bands are found in place of a complete long process of the incus and stapedial crura (Figure 14-24).

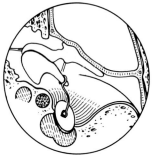

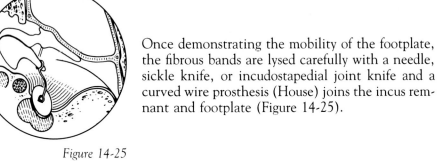

Figure 14-25

Once demonstrating the mobility of the footplate, the fibrous bands are lysed carefully with a needle, sickle knife, or incudostapedial joint knife and a curved wire prosthesis (House) joins the incus remnant and footplate (Figure 14-25).

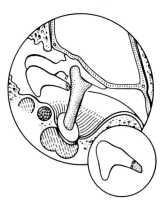

Figure 14-26

A sculptured malleus may bridge the gap (Figure 14-26). Note that the incus remnant is used for support of the homograft malleus.

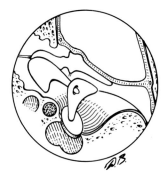

Figure 14-27

A homograft incus may be used to reestablish ossicular continuity (Figure 14-27). This technique fenestrates the homograft incus and is quite difficult for the inexperienced surgeon.

Monopod Stapes

The suprastructure of the stapes is represented by a thickened fibrous band or single crura referred to as a *monopod stapes* (Figure 14-28).

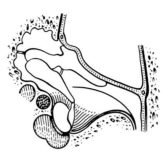

Figure 14-28

The monopod stapes footplate is determined to be mobile. In the case depicted in Figure 14-29 a fenestrated incus homograft has been used (after Marquet).

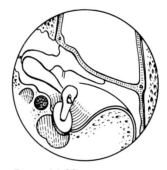

Figure 14-29

Cartilage with perichondrium may be used to buttress the monopod suprastructure. Once placed, the support is packed with Gelfoam to avoid dislocation of the graft in the early postoperative period (Figure 14-30).

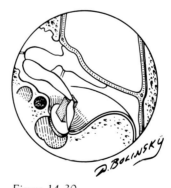

Figure 14-30

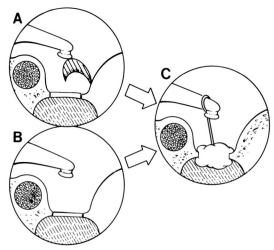

Figure 14-31

Subtotal and Total Absence of Suprastructure

The stapes suprastructure may be subtotally absent and defined only by a thin bony attachment to the lenticular process of the incus (Figure 14-31A). The extreme case would be complete absence of the stapes suprastructure (Figure 14-31B). Management of these stapes anomalies is the same. Mobility of the footplate and absence of the inflammation in the middle-ear space must be ensured. The footplate is removed as in standard stapedectomy, and a fat wire Schuknecht prosthesis is placed (Figure 14-31C). Fat may be obtained from the lobule and (0.004 or 0.005; 38-, 36-g stainless steel wire) is employed. The technique for fashioning the prosthesis is shown in Chapter 9.

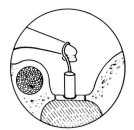

Figure 14-32

A stapedotomy may be performed with placement of a Teflon wire piston (Figure 14-32).

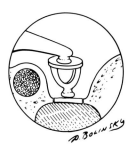

Figure 14-33

An inverted stapes homograft may be used as shown in Figure 14-33. Technical difficulty may be encountered by the novice otologist.

Congenital Fixation

Congenital fixation of the stapes may be differentiated from acquired fixation by history, age of the patient, onset of symptoms, and degree of disability (Figure 14-34).

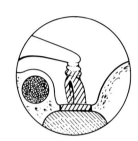

Figure 14-34

The suprastructure is removed and the footplate is "drilled out" (Figure 14-35). The drilling on the footplate should be kept to a minimum, and the burr (diamond) should be kept cool to avoid thermal trauma concomitant to the vibrating trauma introduced. The footplate should be saucerized.

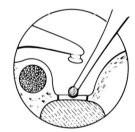

Figure 14-35

Once a stapedotomy is performed, a Teflon wire prosthesis is placed (Figure 14-36). The reader is referred to Chapter 9 on techniques employed in stapes surgery.

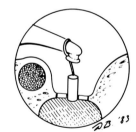

Figure 14-36

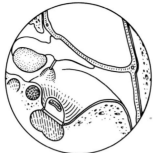

Figure 14-37

Partial Absence of Incudostapedial Complex

Absence of the long process of the incus and stapes suprastructure is shown in Figure 14-37.

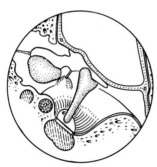

Figure 14-38

A sculptured malleus may be used (homograft) (Figure 14-38).

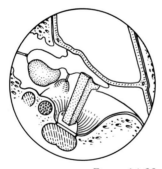

Figure 14-39

A cartilage columella with perichondrium may bridge the defect (Figure 14-39).

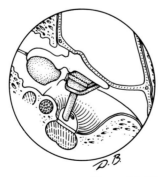

Figure 14-40

A TORP, with partial manubrium and partial tympanic membrane contact, is shown in Figure 14-40. Note the cartilage sandwich between the TORP and the tympanic membrane. This will decrease the chance for extrusion.

Absence of Incus

Congenital absence of the incus with a dehiscent facial nerve is shown in Figure 14-41.

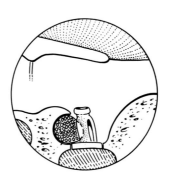

Figure 14-41

The footplate is palpated and a sculptured malleus homograft placed on the inferior surface of the footplate working away from the dehiscent nerve (Figure 14-42).

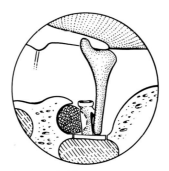

Figure 14-42

A TORP may be used as in 14-42 instead of a malleus homograft. In Figure 14-43 again note the cartilage sandwich as described in Figure 14-40.

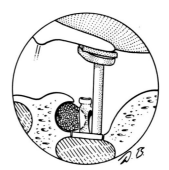

Figure 14-43

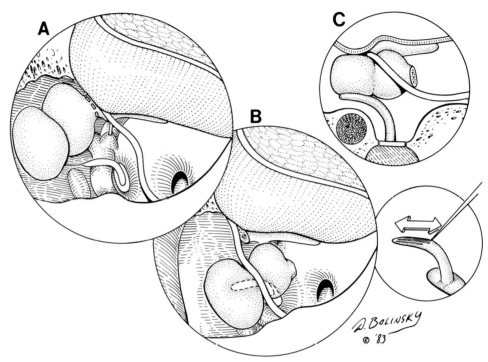

Figure 14-44

Multiple Complex Anomalies

Multiple complex anomalies are demonstrated by the epitympanic fixation of the malleus and incus heads (Figure 14-44A). The long process of the incus is absent, and a fibrous band and partial osseus mass represent the attachment of the incus to the stapes footplate.

The incudomalleolar complex is detached from the epitympanum (Figure 14-44B). The osseus remnant is scored to promote fibrosis as shown in the insert to Figure 14-44B. The incudomalleolar complex is carefully placed on the monopod stapes suprastructure and juxtaposed to the membrane (Figure 14-44C). The chorda tympani is used as a supporting element. Gelfoam packing is carefully placed in the middle ear.

CONGENITAL ABSENCE
OF OVAL WINDOW

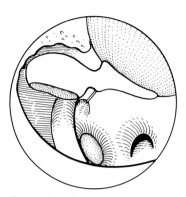

Figure 14-45

VESTIBULOTOMY

Congenital absence of the oval window (Figure 14-45) may be prudentially treated by hearing aids only, fenestration of the horizontal canal, and creation of a new oval window.*

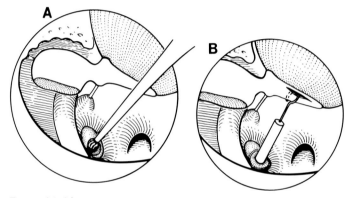

Figure 14-46

The facial nerve is explored (Figure 14-46A). The vestibule is fenestrated and a malleus-to-oval window teflon wire prosthesis placed (Figure 14-46B).

A fat-wire prosthesis may be employed (Figure 14-47).

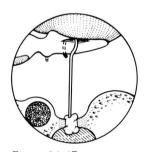

Figure 14-47

A TORP may be employed (Figure 14-48).

*Of all the procedures discussed, this may be the one fraught with the most potential for complication. There are few otologists who can perform with the expertise demonstrated by R. Jahrsdoerfer, M.D., and this should be kept in mind before undertaking the procedure.

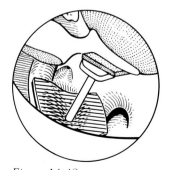

Figure 14-48

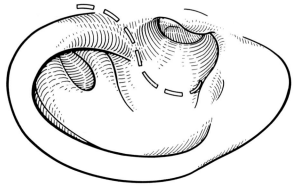

Figure 14-49

FENESTRATION OF HORIZONTAL SEMICIRCULAR CANAL

Following the satisfactory instillation of local anesthetic, a standard endaural incision is made (Figure 14-49).

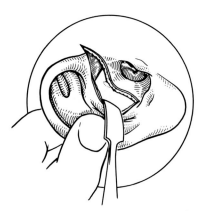

Figure 14-50

With the use of a Lempert periosteal elevator, the auricular skin is reflected posteriorly as the periosteum is elevated, giving exposure to the mastoid cortex (Figure 14-50).

Retractors are placed, exposing the bone overlying the mastoid cortex. In Figure 14-51 note that canal incisions have been made in the tympanosquamous and tympanomastoid suture lines to permit the elevation of a canal skin flap posterior-superiorly, which will be pedicled in the inferior direction.

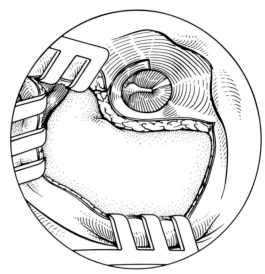

Figure 14-51

Posterior canal wall skin is shown in figure 14-52 to be elevated and reflected in an inferior-anterior direction. With the use of a cutting burr and identifying the spine of Henle, the antrum is opened. Note (in Figure 14-52) that there is no need in the absence of inflammation or infection to open the mastoid widely.

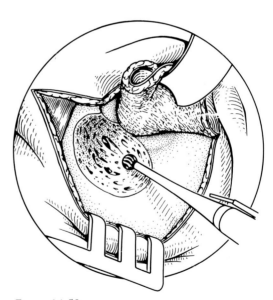

Figure 14-52

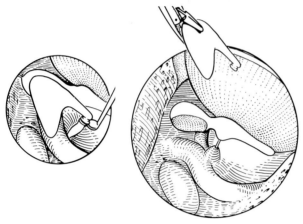

Figure 14-53

The ossicles have been identified (Figure 14-53). To avoid trauma to the inner ear, the tympano-meatal flap is reflected anteriorly, and an incudo-stapedial joint knife separates the lenticular process of the incus from the capitulum of the stapes. The incus is then atraumatically removed.

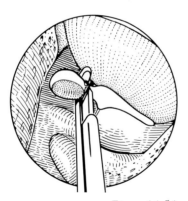

Figure 14-54

The head of the malleus is detached from the manubrium with a malleus nipper (Figure 14-54). Prior to this, the tensor tympani tendon may be severed along with the anterior malleolar ligament. Care should be taken not to violate the tympanic membrane.

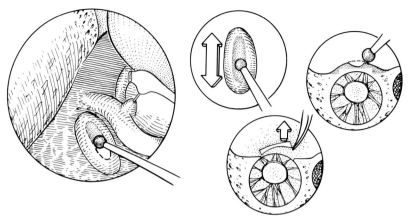

Figure 14-55

The horizontal semicircular canal is identified. As demonstrated in the inserts to Figure 14-55, a diamond burr is used to blue-line the canal down to a thin layer of bone, which then may be gently elevated off the horizontal canal. The surgeon should at all times be aware of the position of the facial nerve.

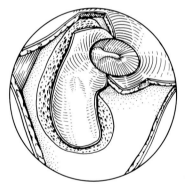

In Figure 14-56 the tympanomeatal flap is rotated and covers the fenestra.

Figure 14-56

Figure 14-57 demonstrates in cross section and surgical position, the placement of the posterior canal wall skin over the fenestra of the horizontal semicircular canal. Note the position of the facial nerve in the cross-sectional view, lying at the level of the horizontal canal fenestration.

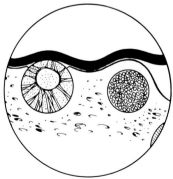

Figure 14-57

CANAL GRAFTING TECHNIQUES

The incisions employed about a rudimentary auricle represent merely one part of a complex series of maneuvers undertaken in the repair of congenital aural atresia. Appreciation of fundamentals of wound healing, scar contracture, tissue devitalization, and flaps must be realized to ensure that the new canal remains patent and that tissue regionally remains available for subsequent auricular reconstruction.

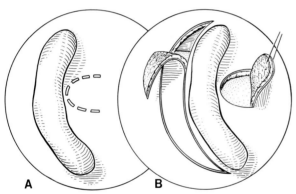

Figure 14-58

CRABTREE'S TECHNIQUE

A U-shaped flap is elevated in the preauricular region several millimeters anterior to the midportion of the auricular remnant. (Figure 14-58A). A postauricular elliptically shaped skin flap is elevated and removed several millimeters posterior to the auricular remnant (Figure 14-58B). This skin is preserved in physiologic solution.

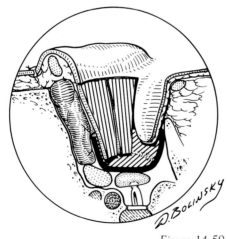

Figure 14-59

Following establishment of a patent canal leading to the middle-ear reconstruction, the anterior flap is laid down along the anterior meatal wall (Figure 14-59). The free skin graft lines the remainder of the canal. The postauricular incision is closed primarily. The mastoid cavity is obliterated with autogenous material (cartilage, muscle, or connective tissue).

LANGE'S TECHNIQUE

An outline is made for a superiorly based transposition flap based on a sloping Z-plasty or S-plasty (Figure 14-60). The auricular remnant is reflected forward while the procedure is performed.

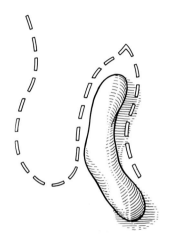

Figure 14-60

Following establishment of a canal, the flap is transposed inferiorly as the auricular remnant is moved posteriorly, and the upper limb of the flap is closed (Figure 14-61). The transposed flap may line the superior and inferior walls of the canal. Free skin flaps will be needed to cover the anterior and posterior meatal walls.

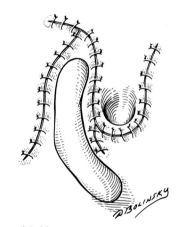

Figure 14-61

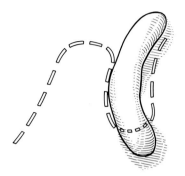

Figure 14-62

ZÜHLKE'S TECHNIQUE

Outline is made for an inferiorly based transposition flap designed with a fundamental Z-plasty or S-plasty technique (see Type II) (Figure 14-62).

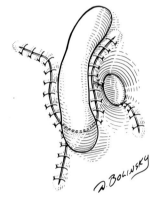

Figure 14-63

The canal is created and the flap transposed (Figure 14-63). Walls not covered by the graft are grafted with split-thickness skin grafts.

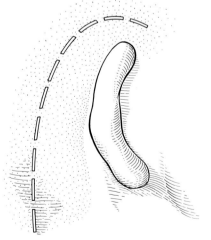

Figure 14-64

MARQUET'S TECHNIQUE

A sloping posterior crescent-shaped incision is made behind the auricular appendage (Figure 14-64). Care must be taken not to cut too deeply for the location of the facial nerve is variable. The flap is undermined anteriorly onto the zygomatic arch.

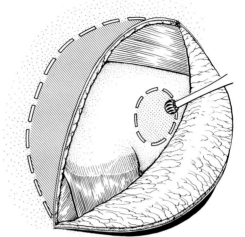

Figure 14-65

The reconstruction is performed with the flap retracted anteriorly (Figure 14-65).

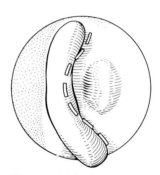

Figure 14-66

Following reconstruction, a counterincision is made along the anterior crease of the auricular appendage, thus creating a bipedicled flap (Figure 14-66).

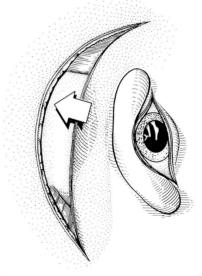

Figure 14-67

The bipedicled flap (with the auricle) is transposed posteriorly, closing the initial incision and leaving the newly created meatus uncovered anteriorly (Figure 14-67).

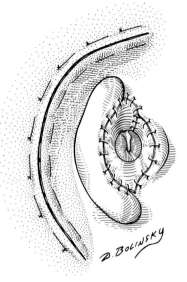

Figure 14-68

Four burr holes are placed in the outer margins of the meatus, and a free skin graft is placed into the meatus and fixed in the technique due to Munster (Figure 14-68). The graft is sutured to the skin at the lateral margins of the canal.

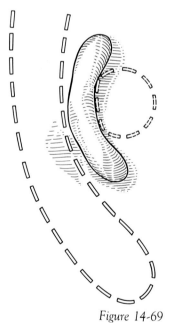

Figure 14-69

LUND AND PHELPS'S TECHNIQUE

A superiorly based random transposition pedicle flap is elevated down posterior to the auricular remnant and liberally extended on to the cervical region. The skin circle outlined anteriorly will be the location of the subsequent canal (Figure 14-69).

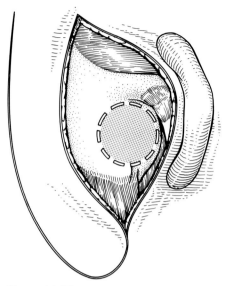

The mastoid cortex, root of the zygoma, and glenoid fossa are exposed anteriorly (Figure 14-70).

Figure 14-70

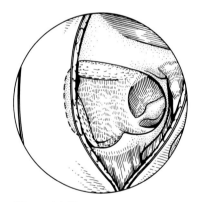

The meatus is opened and the canal created. Middle-ear reconstruction is performed (Figure 14-71).

Figure 14-71

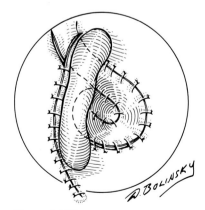

The pedicle is brought into the mastoid cavity and used to line the canal (Figure 14-72). The incision is closed posteriorly in primary fashion.

Figure 14-72

FACIAL NERVE ANOMALIES

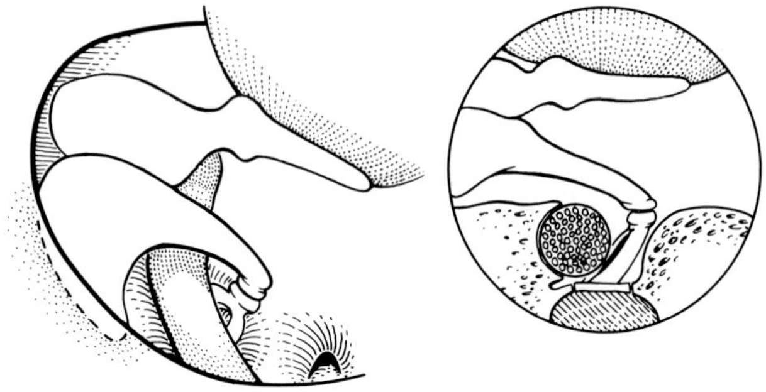

Facial nerve anomalies in ears with congenital anomalies may present an additional surgical challenge to the otologist. This figure demonstrates the horizontal portion of the facial nerve in a dehiscent position overlying the stapes suprastructure. The insert to Figure 14-73 shows a cross section of the dehiscent nerve overlying the footplate superiorly. The suprastructure is noted to be displaced somewhat inferiorly toward the promontory. In cases such as these, careful manipulation around the nerve will sometimes permit reconstruction of the sound conducting mechanism. Some surgeons may attempt to mobilize the nerve superiorly to obtain better exposure (Jahrsdoerfer[6]).

Figure 14-73

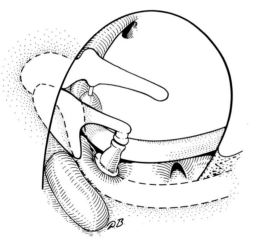

The nerve is noted to take an aberrant course through the middle ear (Figure 14-74). Recognition of the location of the nerve in this position is critical in successful restoration of the ossicular chain without damaging the nerve. Note in Figure 14-74 that the nerve runs anterior to the deformed stapes, oval window, and round window.

Figure 14-74

The nerve is bipedicled about the stapes (Figure 14-75). Although challenging, work on the stapes may be performed.

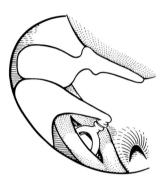

Figure 14-75

A small fenestra stapedotomy with Teflon wire piston permits the reconstruction of the hearing mechanism without harm to the nerve (Figure 14-76).

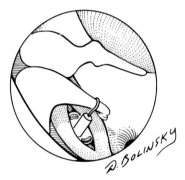

Figure 14-76

DISCUSSION

PSYCHOSOCIAL DILEMMA

Parents faced with the rearing of a child with a significant cosmetic and concomitant sensory deficit may feel strongly obliged to have the child's problems corrected, even in cases where it is not in the best interests of the child from a surgical point of view. We have found that the most reliable way to mollify the fears and anxieties of parents whose children have unilateral auricular anomalies along with congenital atresia is by encouraging their participation in multimodality group discussions. Included among the professionals whose role it will be to educate and support the families are the plastic surgeon, the otologist, the child psychologist, the social worker, the nursing staff, the audiologist, and the speech therapist. Through this multidisciplinary approach, the child's early education and speech training, along with auditory amplification is ensured, and parental anxieties and fears are assuaged.

COSMETIC SURGERY PRIOR TO OTOLOGIC SURGERY?

In unilateral atresia the reconstruction of the external ear and canal prior to the surgical correction for the conductive hearing loss is recommended. The child, when old enough to participate in de-cision-making processes with understanding, can then participate in the latter decision regarding otologic reconstruction. In cases of bilateral atresia, we feel that exploration between the ages of 2 and 4 years on one side should be undertaken by the otologist prior to auricular reconstructions.

The otologist and the plastic surgeon *should* work together closely and consult each other with regard to the approach, the timing, and the order of the surgical procedures so that the best possible cosmetic and functional results can be achieved.

PROSTHETIC AURICLE VERSUS PLASTIC AURICULAR RECONSTRUCTION

With the family and patient prepared to undergo a series of operative procedures over a several-year period, it is our feeling that auricular reconstruction is preferable to prosthesis placement. The otologist working in concert with the plastic surgeon will ensure that minimal trauma is directed against the tissues in the immediate vicinity of the auricle or remnant. Adherence to fundamental plastic surgical tenets regarding wound healing, tissue manipulation, and local flap creation will ensure that the reconstructed auricle manifests near normal color, contour, and consistency; for as Edgerton[4] notes, "size, level, projection, and color and tilt of the ear are more important than details of the helix, antihelix, and cavum."

REFERENCES

1. Bellucci, R. J.: Congenital Aural Malformations—Diagnosis and Treatment. *Otolaryngol. Clin. N. Am.,* 14(1):95–124, 1981.
2. Crabtree, J. A.: Tympanoplastic Techniques in Congenital Atresia. *Arch. Otolaryngol.,* 88:63–70, 1968.
3. Derlacki, E. L.: Surgery for Congenital Atresia. In: Otolaryngology, Vol. I, G. M. English (Ed.). Harper & Row, New York, chap. 13, 1981.
4. Edgerton, M. T.: Ear Construction in Children with Congenital Atresia and Stenosis. *Plast. Reconst. Surg.,* 43(4):373–380, 1969.
5. Jahrsdoerfer, R. A.: Congenital Atresia of the Ear. *Laryngoscope,* 88:1–48, 1978.
6. Jahrsdoerfer, R. A.: Congenital Malformations of the Ear Analysis of 94 Operations. *Ann. Otol.,* 89:348–352, 1980.
7. Lange, G. and Kamgang P.: Erfahrungen der Freiburger HNO-Klinik bei der Behandlung von Ohratresien; Bericht uber 51 Verlaufsbeobachtungen.

Arch. Ohren. Nasen u. Kehlkoph, Heilk., 204:217, 1973.

8. Lund, W. S. and Phelps, P. D.: The Surgery of Congenital Deafness. *J. Laryngol. Otol.*, 92:561–579, 1978.

9. Mundnich, K.: Congenital Abnormalities of the Ear. *Proc. Roy. Soc. Med. Lond.*, 67:1197–1206, 1974.

10. Mundnich, K.: Operations for Congenital Anomalies of the Ear. In: Head and Neck Surgery: Indications, Techniques, Pitfalls, Vol. 3, H. H. Naumann (Ed.). Ear, Saunders, Philadelphia, Chap. 8, 1982.

11. Nager, G. T. and Levin, L. S.: Congenital Aural Atresia: Embryology, Pathology, Classification, Genetics and Surgical Management. In: Otolaryngology, Vol. II, The Ear, Paparella and Shumrick (Eds.). Saunders, Philadelphia, pp. 1303–1344, 1980.

12. Pulec, J. L. and Freedmon, H. M.: Management of Congenital Ear Abnormalities. *Laryngoscope*, 88: 420–434, 1978.

13. Shambaugh, G. E. and Glasscock, M. E., III.: Surgery of the Ear, 3rd ed., Saunders, Philadelphia, 1980.

14. Schuknecht, H. F.: Reconstructive Procedures for Congenital Aural Atresia. *Arch. Otolaryngol.*, 101: 170–172, 1975.

15. Schwaber, M. K., Glasscock, M. E. III, Nissen, A. J., and Jackson, C. G.: The Place of Fenestration in Congenital Ear Surgery. *Am. J. Otol.*, 4:222–225, 1983.

16. Tanzer, R. C.: Microtia. *Clin. Plast. Surg.*, 5(3): 317–336, 1978.

17. Zühlke, D.: Chirurgische Behandlung der Missbildungen des Ohres. *Arch. klin. exp. Ohren. Nasen u. Kehlkoph Heilk.*, 202:153, 1972.

II

Neuro-otology
Gale Gardner

15

Balance Disorders
——of Labyrinthine Origin——

Balance disorders resulting from labyrinthine dysfunction of multiple etiology frequently respond to nonsurgical management. When they do not, and when the symptoms are significant, surgery may be indicated. The surgical approaches that may be employed are divided into two groups: those used when useful hearing has been lost and those used when useful hearing is present.

SURGICAL MANAGEMENT WHEN USEFUL HEARING HAS BEEN LOST

TRANSMASTOID LABYRINTHECTOMY

Under general anesthesia, supplemented by infiltrative anesthesia containing epinephrine, an in-

cision is made either in the postauricular fold or 1 cm posterior to it. The incision extends in depth to the level of the temporalis fascia (Figure 15-1).

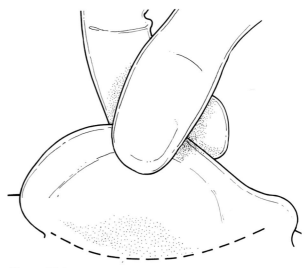

Figure 15-1

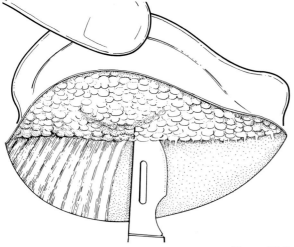

The auricle is lifted away from the scalp, and by using either a scalpel or cutting cautery, the soft tissue is elevated (Figure 15-2).

Figure 15-2

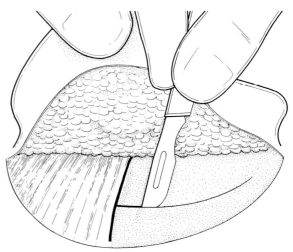

Figure 15-3

Incisions are made through the periosteum, first along the linea temporalis at the lower margin of the temporalis muscle and then perpendicular to this over the surface of the mastoid process to the mastoid tip (Figure 15-3).

A periosteal elevator is used to elevate the periosteum posteriorly, superiorly, and anteriorly (Figure 15-4).

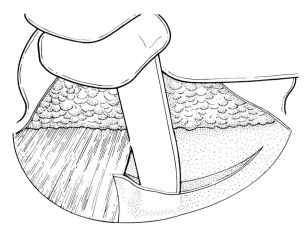

Figure 15-4

Retractors are placed. With the use of a high-speed surgical drill, either electrically or air driven, and with continuous irrigation and suction, the mastoid cortex is removed (Figure 15-5). The cribriform area and the linea temporalis are identified, and initial bone cuts are made parallel to the superior and posterior margins of the external auditory canal.

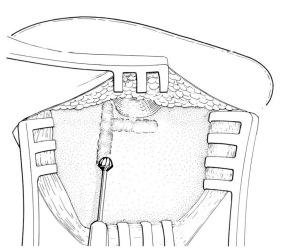

Figure 15-5

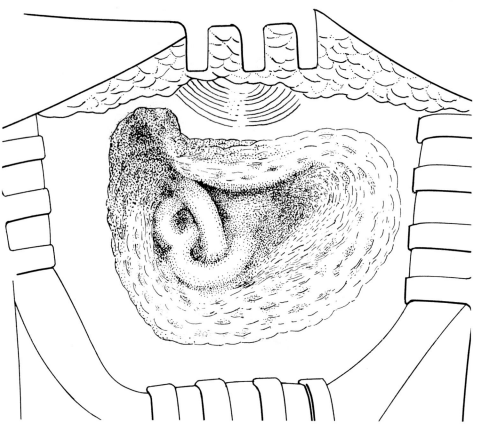

Figure 15-6

The mastoid cortex is removed so as to create a bowl with no overhanging margins (Figure 15-6). The middle and posterior fossa plates are skeletonized, as is the vertical or mastoid segment of the facial nerve. The otic capsule bone of the three semicircular canals is identified. This portion of the operation is ordinarily best performed with a sharp cutting burr.

By use of the same technique, with a smaller cutting burr and smaller-caliber irrigation suction unit, the horizontal canal is opened (Figure 15-7). It is important for the operating surgeon to be assured that the correct ear is indeed being operated on before this step is taken. The incus may be removed at this time.

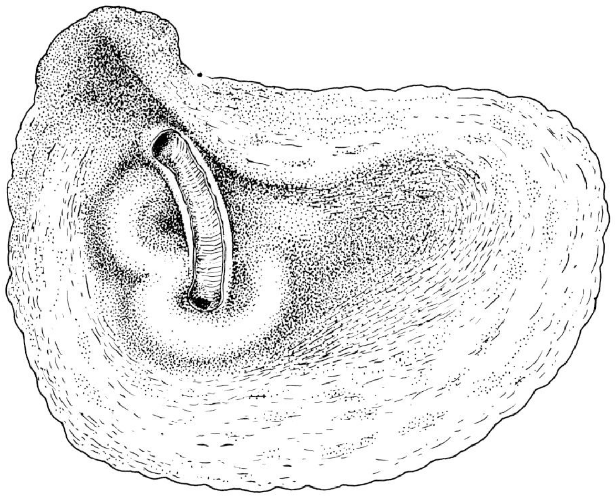

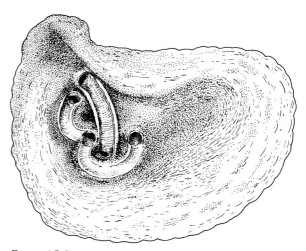

Figure 15-7

With the use of a systematic technique that is comfortable for the surgeon, the remaining two canals are opened with the cutting burr (Figure 15-8). The author prefers to extend the horizontal cut posteriorly until the posterior canal is exposed. The posterior canal is then opened inferiorly, working medially to the facial nerve. It is then followed superiorly as it loops anteriorly into the common crus, which is followed superiorly and anteriorly into the superior canal, which is in turn followed anteriorly to its ampulla, adjacent to the ampulla of the horizontal canal, which is also located anteriorly. A diamond burr may be used to control bleeding and, in fact, whenever the surgeon is more comfortable with it.

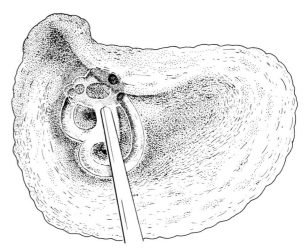

Figure 15-8

The remaining bone of the horizontal canal is removed and the bone covering the tympanic segment of the facial nerve skeletonized in order to allow wide opening of the vestibule (Figure 15-9). The three ampullae, the utricle, and the saccule are identified directly. To avoid failure, the membranous end organs must be completely removed. It is important to avoid injury to the facial nerve during this step of the procedure. The operation is completed by placing segments of temporalis muscle into the vestibule. The mastoid bowl is filled with moist Gelfoam, the wound is closed routinely in layers without drainage, and a mastoid dressing is placed.

Figure 15-9

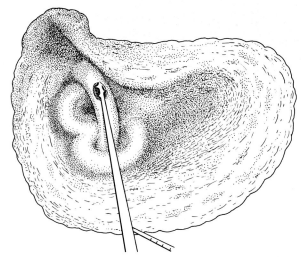

Figure 15-10

ALTERNATIVE PROCEDURES

Day Procedure[10]

Only the horizontal semicircular canal was opened, and a coagulating current was applied to a probe placed near the ampulla (Figure 15-10).

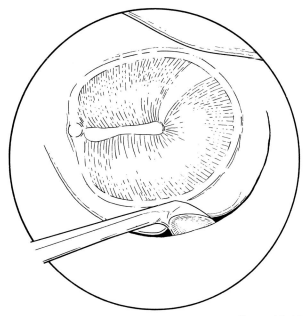

Transcanal Labyrinthectomy[8,27]

A tympanomeatal flap is elevated as shown in Figure 15-11.

Figure 15-11

Bone is curetted away from the posterior superior canal wall, exposing the stapes (Figure 15-12).

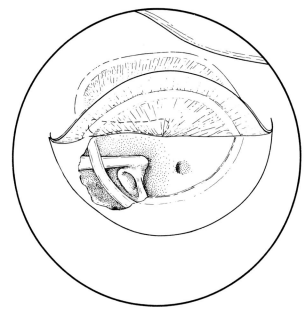

Figure 15-12

The incudostapedial joint is incised, and the stapes arch and footplate are removed (Figure 15-13).

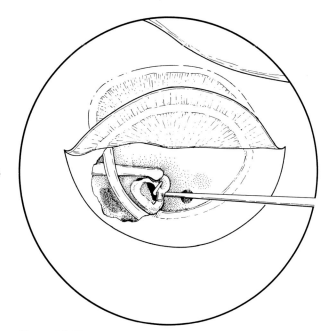

Figure 15-13

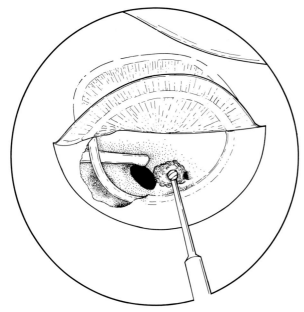

A handpiece with burr designed for the ear canal is used to drill away the bone between the oval and round windows (Figure 15-14).

Figure 15-14

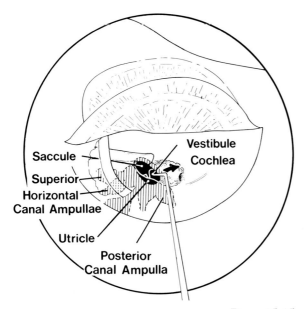

The drawing in Figure 15-15 is based on an illustration by Anson and Donaldson[2] and relates the transcanal procedure to the underlying structures within the labyrinth. A working knowledge of the anatomy is critical to successful removal of the membranous labyrinthine end organs. Complete removal of the membranous end organs is essential.

Figure 15-15

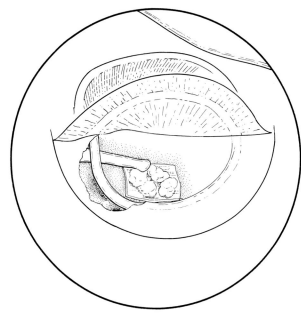

Following removal of the membranous end organs,Gelfoam soaked with gentamicin, streptomycin, or alcohol may be placed within the vestibule and temporalis fascia placed over the bony opening (Figure 15-16).

Figure 15-16

Translabyrinthine Nerve Section (House[17])

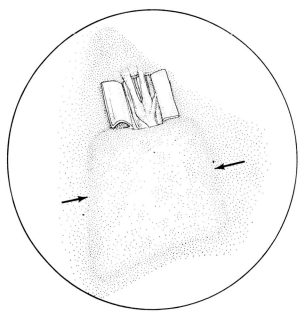

In the case illustrated in Figure 15-17 a simple mastoidectomy has been performed and the bone of the labyrinth removed so as to skeletonize the dura of the internal auditory canal (dura has been incised, exposing the vestibular nerve) and the dura overlying the posterior fossa (see arrows). For a more detailed view of this exposure, see Figures 17-11 and 17-12. Note the superior vestibular nerve on the left, the much smaller nerve to the posterior semicircular canal on the right, and the intervening inferior vestibular nerve. Note that the most peripheral fibers of the nerve lie on a bony surface that is the vertical crest of the internal auditory canal ("Bill's bar") and directly beneath which (medially) lies the facial nerve.

Figure 15-17

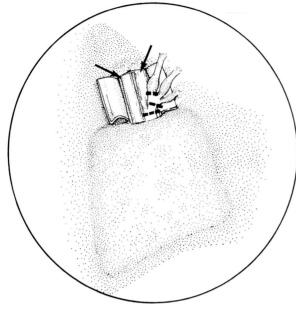

Figure 15-18 shows that the superior vestibular nerve has been lifted away from the facial nerve (see left arrow), with the inferior vestibular nerve and the nerve to the posterior canal. The cochlear division (see right arrow) is seen "beneath" (medial to) the vestibular grouping of nerves. Nerve sectioning is now performed. Great care must be taken to avoid injury to the facial nerve, or to the vasculature of the canal, which may include a loop of the anterior inferior cerebellar artery. Depending on the preference of the surgeon, one may section only the superior vestibular nerve (upper divided line), the entire vestibular nerve (middle divided line), or the entire eighth nerve, including the cochlear division (lower divided line). Note that the cuts are made central to the ovoid swelling that represents Scarpa's ganglion. Adequate exposure should be available to see the anatomy clearly. Sharp, specially designed microscissors are desirable.

Figure 15-18

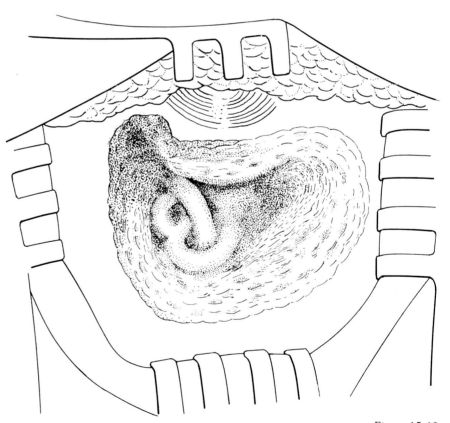

Figure 15-19

SURGICAL MANAGEMENT WHEN USEFUL HEARING IS PRESENT

MÉNIÈRE'S DISEASE

Endolymphatic Sac Subarachnoid Shunt (House,[18] Based on Work of Portmann[25])

A simple mastoidectomy is performed, with skeletonizing of the posterior fossa dura and the mastoid segment of the facial nerve (Figure 15-19).

The endolymphatic sac is identified, based on the fact that the endolymphatic duct (which forms the posterior superior margin of the sac) exits from beneath the posterior semicircular canal at a nearly invariable location, since this is at the junction of the posterior one-third and the inferior one-third of the canal (Figure 15-20). The sac is identified by gently depressing the dura away from the overlying bone of the posterior canal and noting the spot at which the dura is fixed to the bone of the canal by the duct. The sac may be relatively inaccessible depending on the proximity of the adjacent anatomic structures, including the facial nerve (which usually overlies the sac in a lateral projection) and the sigmoid sinus and jugular bulb, both of which may "crowd" the sac and even overlie it; the sigmoid sinus from a lateral projection as shown in Figure 15-20; and the bulb from an inferior projection.

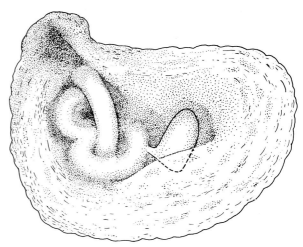

Figure 15-20

To overcome these problems, when they exist, it is necessary to skeletonize each of these structures. Exposure of the facial nerve allows access to the sac medial to the nerve, whereas exposure of the sigmoid sinus (shown in Figure 15-21) and jugular bulb allows decompression of either or both of these structures with bone wax, thereby allowing visualization of the sac. The bone wax is removed following the procedure.

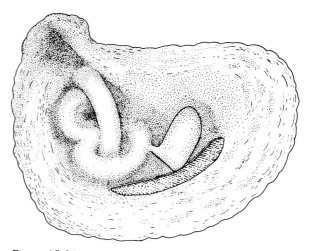

Figure 15-21

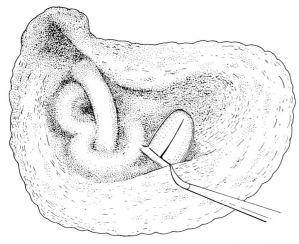

Figure 15-22

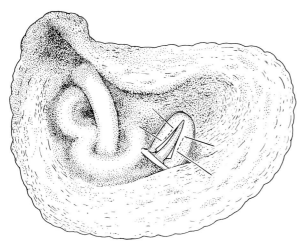

Figure 15-23

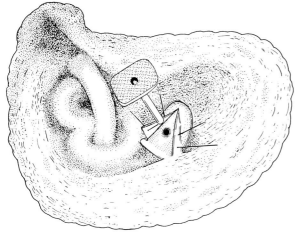

Figure 15-24

After the sac is adequately exposed, a T-shaped incision is made through the outer dural wall of the sac (Figure 15-22). Care must be taken actually to enter the smooth, glistening interior of the sac, and not to penetrate prematurely through the medial sac wall into the posterior fossa.

With the use of a double-armed 5-0 silk suture material with specially designed finely curved dural needles, sutures are placed through both dural edges, and the needles are then brought externally (Figure 15-23). The two needles are then passed through the opposing edges of a segment of vein taken from the antecubital fossa of the arm, the needle entering the vein from the serosal surface and exiting from the adventitial surface. The needles are then tagged and set aside.

An opening is then made in the medial dural wall of the sac, exposing the underlying arachnoid, which produces a dark bubble (Figure 15-24). A silastic shunt tube having an acute angle between the flange and the tube of between 30°–45° is then bluntly inserted through the arachnoid "bubble" into the subarachnoid space. It is important that the shunt tube be held in such a way that the tip is directed anteriorly and superiorly rather than medially, posteriorly, or inferiorly (into the cerebellum). This is a particularly critical part of the operation, as damage to an adjacent blood vessel may produce significant bleeding, and rarely disastrous results. A surgeon who has not gained clear-cut control of the anatomy should consider an alternative procedure that does not require entry into the subarachnoid space. If the shunt tube can be safely placed, however, the flange is next seated securely within the sac lumen.

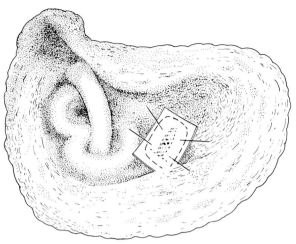

The vein is then lowered into position over the sac and sutured in place, with the intimal surface placed medially (Figure 15-25).

Figure 15-25

Other Endolymphatic Sac Procedures

Sac decompression (Shambaugh[30]).   A simple mastoidectomy is performed, and the endolymphatic sac exposed (Figure 15-26), as previously illustrated in Figures 15-19, 15-20, and 15-21. Using this procedure, Shambaugh demonstrated results approximating these obtained with other procedures. In a much smaller-scale experience, the author failed to achieve comparable results with decompression, and the procedure was abandoned.

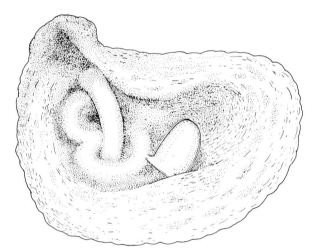

Mastoid shunt (Arenberg,[3] Morrison,[21] Shea[31]). The sac is exposed, the external dural covering incised, and drainage established into the mastoid (Figure 15-27). Shea used Teflon film, as shown in Figure 15-27, extending from the sac into the mastoid space. Not shown here are Arrenberg's technique of placement of a one-way valve into the endolymphatic duct with Silastic sheeting extending into the mastoid, and Morrison's use of a capillary tube inserted into the duct and connecting to a Silastic sponge brought out into the mastoid space.

Figure 15-26

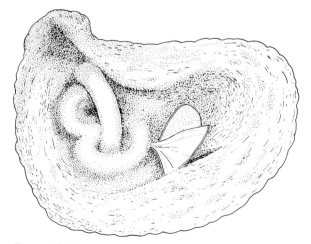

Figure 15-27

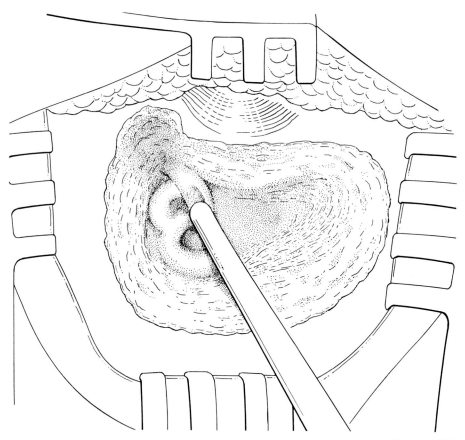

Figure 15-28

Ultrasound, transmastoid (Altman and Waltner,[1] *Arslan,*[4] *Pennington,*[23]*).* The mastoid cavity has been opened and the ultrasonic probe placed against the thinned horizontal semicircular canal (Figure 15-28). Ultrasonic waves are thus applied to the labyrinth.

Cryosurgery, transmastoid (Wolfson[35]*).* A cryosurgical probe is placed against the thinned horizontal canal as shown in Figure 15-28.

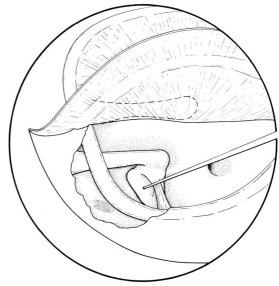

Decompression of the labyrinth (Fick[11]). A sharp pick is used to penetrate first the stapes footplate, and then the saccule (Figure 15-29). This procedure is mentioned as being of historical interest only; it does not provide effective relief of symptoms with preservation of hearing.

Figure 15-29

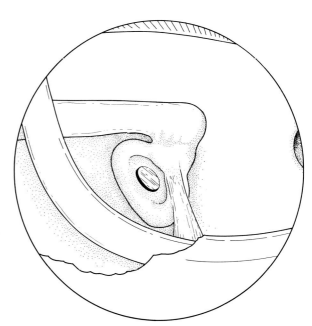

Tack procedure (Cody[9]). A stainless-steel tack has been inserted into the vestibule through a hole made in the footplate, allowing puncture of the underlying saccule (Figure 15-30). This procedure is less traumatic than Fick's and allows repetitive saccular decompression. Cody continues to find it useful. Precise instrumentation following Cody's recommended technique is important.

Figure 15-30

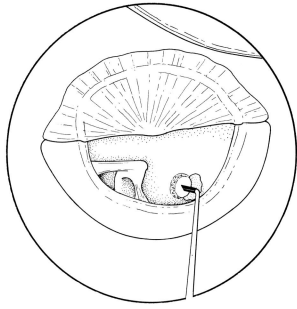

Otic-perotic shunt (House,[19] Pulec[6]). After exposure of the middle-ear space, the round window niche is exposed by removal of overlying bone as necessary. Pulec described elevation of a mucous membrane flap from the round-window membrane. A platinum shunt tube is shown in Figure 15-31 being introduced through the membrane toward the stapes, with the intent of placing it through the basilar membrane and thereby connecting the scala media and scala tympani. The flap is replaced and covered with Gelfoam. (House discontinued use of this procedure after noting a 20 percent incidence of additional hearing loss. Note that the concept reappeared in the early 1980s.)

Figure 15-31

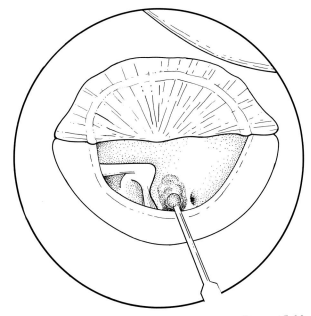

Cryosurgery of the promontory (House[19]). A dental drill is used to thin the bone of the promontory between the oval and round windows (Figure 15-32).

Figure 15-32

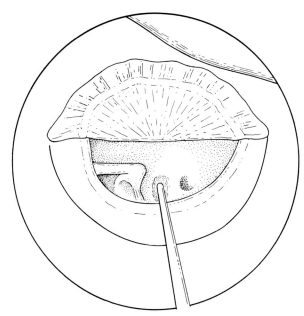

A Cooper cryosurgical probe is now applied to the thinned area of the promontory, with the intent of producing a lesion in the wall of the saccule, thereby allowing release of endolymph from the scala media into the scala tympani (Figure 15-33). Facial paralysis and tympanic membrane perforations occurred postoperatively. House discontinued use of this procedure.

Figure 15-33

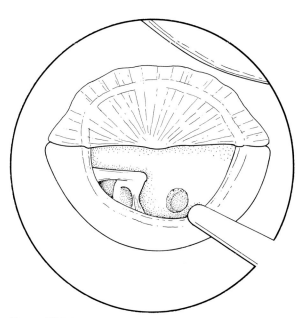

Round-window ultrasonic irradiation (Basek,[7] Kossoff,[20] Pennington[24]). The middle ear is exposed, and a small diamond burr is used to drill away the superior lip of the round-window niche (Figure 15-34). The ultrasonic probe is being positioned into the niche. The probe must be immersed in saline during the procedure, and care must be taken to maintain the probe tip in a fixed position in the niche, with the tip directed away from the facial nerve.

Figure 15-34

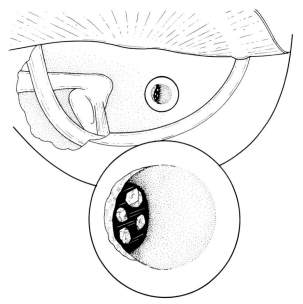

Figure 15-35

Round-window application of sodium chloride crystals (Arslan[5]). The round-window niche is visualized (Figure 15-35, as previously illustrated in Figure 15-31). Sterilized sodium chloride crystals no larger than 1 mm in size are placed in the round-window niche, filling it. Although Arslan reported good results with this procedure, it has not gained frequent use and is not recommended by the author.

Cochleosacculotomy, cochleostomy (Morrison,[22] Schuknecht[29]). Schuknecht has described insertion of a 3-mm right-angled pick through the exposed round window membrane, the osseous spiral lamina, and the dilated cochlear duct, into the saccule at the level of the footplate. On removal of the pick, the round-window niche is packed with moist Gelfoam. Morrison has referred to a similar procedure, in which he punctures the cochlear partition of the basilar coil of the cochlea.

Comment. These procedures are still in the investigative stage and require a longer period of follow-up before their values can be determined.

BENIGN PAROXYSMAL POSITIONAL VERTIGO

Singular Neurectomy (Gacek[12])

The middle ear has been exposed, with a very small burr used to drill an oval-shaped defect in the bony floor of the round window niche (Figure 15-36).

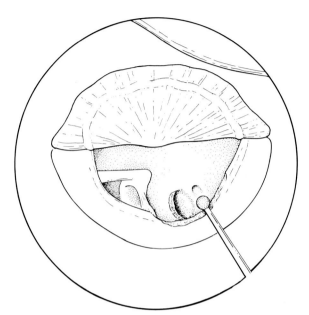

Figure 15-36

At a depth of approximately 1.5–2 mm, the nerve to the posterior semicircular canal is seen in Figure 15-37 as a white, linear structure and is elevated with a right-angled hook.

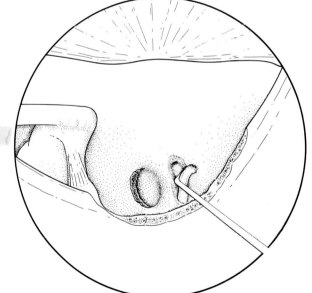

Figure 15-37

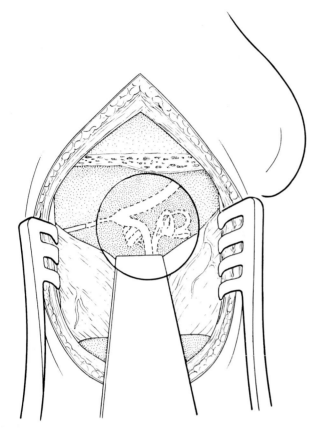

Figure 15-38

INCAPACITATING VERTIGO OF MULTIPLE CAUSE

Middle Fossa Vestibular Nerve Section (House[16])

The patient is under general anesthesia. The surgeon operates from the head of the table. In Figure 15-38 the right ear is exposed, with the face turned to the left. A skin incision has been made one fingerbreadth anterior to the tragus, extending from the natural hairline superiorly 3–4 inches. Deep incisions have been made through the temporalis muscle vertically and along the linea temporalis horizontally. A craniotomy has been performed, using a cutting burr so as to preserve the block of bone that is outlined. The block measures 3 cm in width, with 2 cm anterior to the midline of the external auditory meatus. The bone block extends vertically from the floor of the middle fossa to the squamoparietal suture line. A House-Urban middle fossa retractor has been placed so as to elevate the temporal lobe. The facial nerve, greater superficial petrosal nerve, cochlear nerve, superior vestibular nerve, and semicircular canals are shown in dotted outline in Figure 15-38.

In Figure 15-39 the same basic structures of the temporal bone are shown ghosted in, as seen from above through this approach.

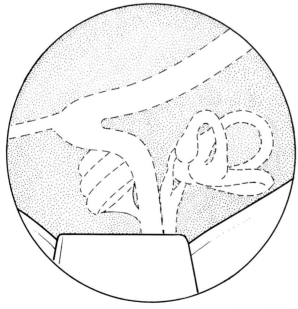

Figure 15-39

By use of continuous suction and irrigating solution for exposure, a diamond burr has been used to drill away the bone overlying the lateral end of the internal auditory canal. The method advocated by Fisch has been employed, in which the superior semicircular canal has first been skeletonized, and an angle of 60° taken from the superior canal, representing the expected location of the internal canal. It is important to expose the extreme lateral end of the canal and to skeletonize the superior vestibular nerve, shown in Figure 15-40 on the right and the facial nerve on the left, with the intervening wedge of bone that represents the vertical crest of the internal auditory canal. The final layer of bone is chipped away and the nerves exposed, as shown. An alternative method of identifying the internal canal is House's technique of skeletonizing the greater superficial petrosal nerve from the facial hiatus to the geniculate ganglion and then following the facial nerve into the internal auditory canal.

As shown in Figure 15-41, the dura of the internal auditory canal has been incised and the most lateral fibers of the superior vestibular nerve elevated. The nerve is sectioned central to Scarpa's ganglion, using specially designed, sharp scissors. An alternative procedure is also to identify and section the inferior vestibular nerve, located immediately beneath the superior nerve and the horizontal crest. The entire vestibular nerve may then be resected at a level central to Scarpa's ganglion.

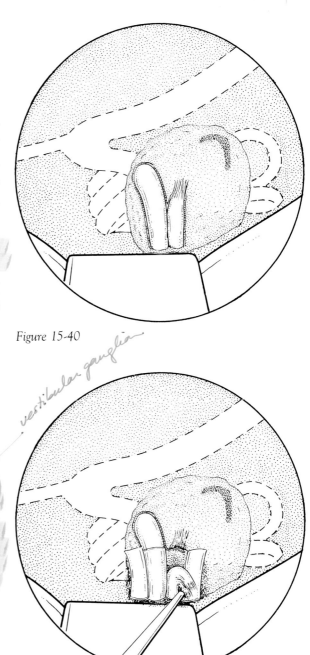

Figure 15-40

vestibular ganglia

Figure 15-41

The wound is closed. Care is taken to close all exposed air cells with bone wax. Temporalis fascia and muscle are placed over the opening in the internal canal, the bone square replaced, and the wound closed in layers. Fisch prefers to drain the wound with continuous suction.

Temporal bone surgery performed through a subtemporal or middle fossa approach (see Figures 15-38–15-41) is extremely demanding and relatively unforgiving of surgical errors. Dealing with the soft-tissue structures of the temporal bone through this approach requires nearly exact control of the angles involved, which necessitates correct positioning of the head, proper placement of skin, soft tissue, and bone cuts. If the skin and subcutaneous incision is carried too far inferiorly, the most superior branch of the facial nerve may be sectioned. If the vertical bone cuts are not kept parallel and properly angled, placement of the middle fossa retractor may be compromised and resulting surgical exposure limited. Initial errors may carry over into failure to identify basic landmarks, which may then result in surgical error such as drilling into the cochlea or damage to the facial nerve. More than in most procedures, middle fossa surgery demands disciplined preoperative experience in the temporal bone dissection laboratory and surgical training in the multitude of details comprising this surgery, relatively few of which can be included in a surgical atlas such as this.

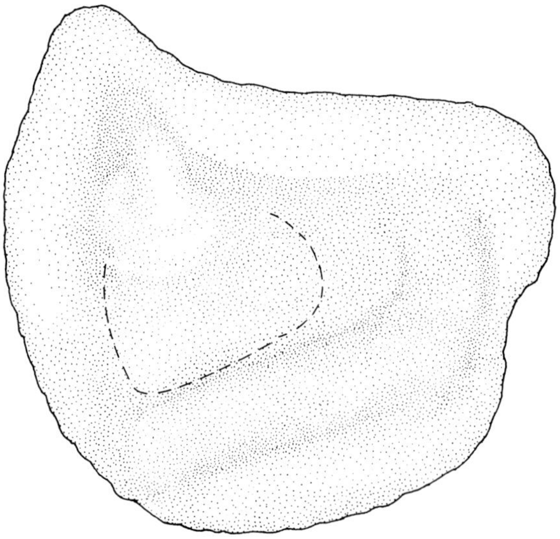

Retrolabyrinthine Nerve Section

After a simple mastoidectomy has been completed, the sigmoid sinus, middle fossa dural plate, and horizontal and posterior semicircular canals are skeletonized. An incision is made through the dura (Figure 15-42) first along a line slightly anterior to the anterior margin of the sigmoid sinus, with care taken to avoid injury to subdural and subarachnoid structures. The incision is then carried anteriorly both (1) inferior and parallel to the superior petrosal sinus (Figure 15-42, superiorly) and (2) superior to the jugular bulb (Figure 15-42, inferiorly). This incision is shown dotted in Figure 15-42 and is designed to contain the endolymphatic sac, in order to avoid its sacrifice.

Figure 15-42

Elevation of the flap exposes (1) the brainstem anteriorly; (2) the cerebellum, which is retracted carefully, posteriorly; and (3) cranial nerves 5 (shown on the extreme left in Figure 15-43), 9–12 (shown as two nerves on the extreme right in Figure 15-43), and 7 and 8 (shown as two nerves in Figure 15-43, center). Of the latter, the more superior nerve closest to the operator should be the superior vestibular nerve, with the facial nerve immediately anterior to it. Those advocating this approach believe that it is possible to separate the fibers of the vestibular division of the eighth cranial nerve from the cochlear fibers. (*Note:* Entry into the subarachnoid space and cerebellopontine angle requires careful technique and should be performed with neurosurgical participation, or availability.)

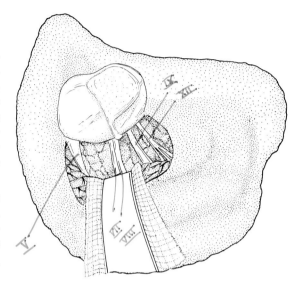

Figure 15-43

REPAIR OF ROUND-WINDOW FISTULA (GOODHILL[14])

The round-window membrane is exposed as shown, with a tympanomeatal flap turned forward. It is usually necessary to remove an overhanging bony lip with a rotating burr. A linear tear is shown in Figure 15-44. The oval window should also be examined closely for a fistula.

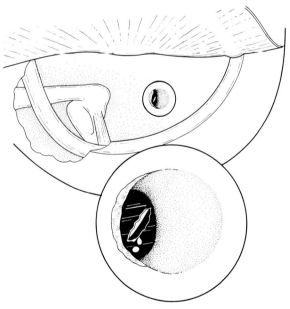

Figure 15-44

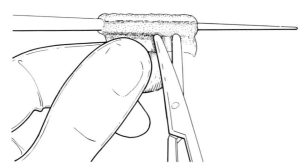

Tissue is obtained for closure of the fistula. Figure 15-45 shows a vein taken from the dorsum of the hand, with the adventitial layer being removed from the vein proper, which is then incised longitudinally. A segment of either adventitia or vein may be approximated against the tear. Goodhill described the use of perichondrium, and fat or fascia are suitable for fistula closure also.

Figure 15-45

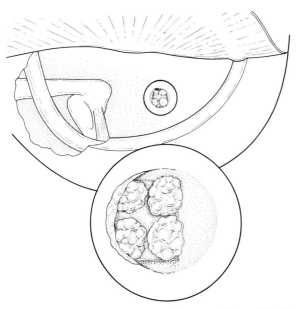

The tissue selected is laid over the round-window membrane, and then covered with tiny pieces of fat, followed by Gelfoam (Figure 15-46).

Figure 15-46

DISCUSSION

The transmastoid labyrinthectomy procedure (Figures 15-1–15-9) allows complete access to the vestibular end organs, yet avoids the potential complications associated with opening of the subarachnoid space. Although the author prefers this procedure, a number of other procedures have been described and advocated for labyrinthine destruction in the absence of useful hearing in the involved ear (Figures 15-10–15-18).

Cawthorne's[8] experience was that the transcanal labyrinthectomy procedure (Figures 15-11–15-16) was a useful one. He felt that it was unnecessary to place an ototoxic substance within the vestibule. Silverstein[32] has extended this procedure to allow access to the internal auditory canal in order to permit partial or total sectioning of the eighth cranial nerve. This is a formidable procedure because of the anatomic limitations.

House has advocated the translabyrinthine nerve section approach (Figures 15-17, 15-18) as the most likely to produce permanent denervation of the vestibular nerve because the nerve may be sectioned central to Scarpa's ganglion, thereby eliminating the possibility of nerve regeneration peripherally from the neuronal cells in the ganglion. Schuknecht,[28] however, has questioned the validity of this, based on experimental evidence using cats. The evidence was less conclusive in two human temporal bones of patients having undergone transcanal labyrinthectomy. The author's experience obtained clinically has been that the results of transmastoid labyrinthectomy and translabyrinthine nerve section are similar, but that both have been superior to transcanal labyrinthectomy, which depends on relatively blind identification of the neural end organs.

The author has slightly modified House's endolymphatic sac subarachnoid shunt procedure (Figures 15-19–15-25) by using (1) an angulated shunt tube that projects the tip of the tube anteriorly into the cerebellopontine angle cistern and (2) vein rather than fascia for sac closure. The reason for the latter is to minimize fibrosis and possible sac obliteration.

The shunt procedure as described has produced reasonably satisfactory results.[13] Nevertheless, this procedure has not gained the universal approval of the otologic community because of less than ideal clinical results and because of theoretical objections raised by Schuknecht and others regarding the relative pressure between endolymph and cerebrospinal fluid (CSF). These reasons, plus the necessity of entering the subarachnoid space, have justified the search for a more satisfactory procedure for solving this problem. As a result, a large number of procedures have been developed (see Figures 15-26–15-35).

Recent reports by Bailey[6] and Tabb[34] indicate a continuing interest in the round-window ultrasonic radiation technique (Figure 15-34). If this procedure is to be employed, careful attention to the exact details of instrumentation and technique are critical to success and avoidance of complications. Electronystagmogram monitoring is recommended.

Gacek recommends probing of the central end of the canal to prevent nerve regeneration. He more recently recommended that bone removal be carried out so as to approach the inferior aspect of the nerve canal and thereby lessen the risk of damage to the cochlea. Gacek pointed out that the singular canal may be located superior to the attachment of the round window membrane, making this surgical procedure impractical in these particular cases. Gacek has pointed out, and the author would like to emphasize, the importance of developing a thorough knowledge of the surgical anatomy that is involved, through temporal bone laboratory dissections.

Regarding the singular neurectomy procedure (Figures 15-36, 15-37), an alternative form of treatment to temporal bone surgery performed through a subtemporal or middle fossa approach is based on the procedure performed by Dandy in the early part of this century. Dandy attempted to section selectively the vestibular fibers of the eighth cranial nerve through a suboccipital approach. In doing this without the type of magnification available today, and perhaps because of limitations involved with the approach, hearing loss was not uncommon postoperatively. Silverstein[33] has proposed that a similar procedure be performed through the retro-labyrinthine approach that Hitselberger[15] developed for tic douloureux surgery. The procedure differs from Dandy's in that the operating microscope is used, and the approach is from anterior to the sigmoid, rather than posteriorly.

REFERENCES

1. Altmann, F. and Waltner, J. G.: The Treatment of Ménière's Disease with Ultrasonic Waves. Arch. Otolaryngol., 69:7–12, 1959.
2. Anson, B. J. and Donaldson, J. A.: The Surgical Anatomy of the Temporal Bone. Saunders, Philadelphia, p. 105, 1967.
3. Arenberg, I. K., Stahle, J., Wilbrand, H., et al.: The Unidirectional Inner Ear Valve Implant for Endolymphatic Sac Surgery in Ménière's Disease. Arch. Otolaryngol., 104:694–704, 1978.
4. Arslan, M.: Treatment of Ménière's Syndrome by Direct Application of Ultra-Sound Waves to the Vestibular System. In: Proceedings of the 5th International Congress of Otolaryngology, Amsterdam, 1953. Assen, Netherlands, 1953.
5. Arslan, M.: Treatment of Ménière's Disease by Apposition of Sodium Chloride Crystals on the Round Window. Laryngoscope, 82:1736–1750, 1972.
6. Bailey, H. A. T. and Pappas, J. J.: Round Window Ultrasonic Irradiation in the Treatment of Ménière's Disease. J. Ark. Med. Soc., 72(10):391–396, 1976.
7. Basek, M.: Treatment of Ménière's Disease with Ultrasound (Round Window Technique). Laryngoscope, 80:768–776, 1970.
8. Cawthorne, T. E.: The Treatment of Ménière's Disease. J. Laryngol. Otol., 58:363–371, 1943.
9. Cody, D., Thane R., Simonton, K. M., et al.: Automatic Repetitive Decompression of the Saccule in Endolymphatic Hydrops (Tack Operation). Laryngoscope, 77:1480–1501, 1967.
10. Day, K. M.: Labyrinth Surgery for Ménière's Disease. Laryngoscope, 53:617–630, 1943.
11. Fick, I. A. van N.: Decompression of the Labyrinth. Arch. Otolaryngol., 79:447–458, 1964.
12. Gacek, R. R.: Transection of the Posterior Ampullary Nerve for the Relief of Benign Paroxysmal Positional Vertigo. Ann. Otol. Rhinol. Laryngol., 83:596–605, 1974.
13. Gardner, G.: Endolymphatic Sac Shunt Operation in Ménière's Disease. Trans. Am. Acad. Ophthalmol. Otolaryngol., 80:306–313, 1975.
14. Goodhill, V.: Sudden Deafness and Round Window Rupture. Laryngoscope, 81:1462–1474, 1971.
15. Hitselberger, W. E. and Pulec, J. L.: Trigeminal Nerve (Posterior Root) Retrolabyrinthine Selective Section. Arch. Otolaryngol., 96:412–415, 1972.
16. House, W. F.: Surgical Exposure of the Internal Auditory Canal and its Contents Through the Middle Cranial Fossa. Laryngoscope, 71:1363–1385, 1961.
17. House, W. F.: Middle Cranial Fossa Approach to the Petrous Pyramid: Report of 50 Cases. Arch. Otolaryngol., 78:460–469, 1963.
18. House, W. F.: Subarachnoid Shunt for Drainage of Hydrops. A Report of 146 Cases. Laryngoscope, 75:1547–1551, 1965.
19. House, W. F.: Cryosurgical Treatment of Ménière's Disease. Arch. Otolaryngol., 84:616–629, 1966.
20. Kossoff, G., Wadsworth, J. H., and Dudley, P. F.: The Round Window Ultrasonic Technique for Treatment of Ménière's Disease. Arch. Otolaryngol., 86:535–542, 1967.
21. Morrison, A. W.: Capillary Endolymphatic Shunt. In: Proceedings of the Sixth Shambaugh International Workshop on Otomicrosurgery and Third Shea Fluctuant Hearing Loss Symposium, G. E. Shambaugh, and J. J. Shea (Eds). Strode, Huntsville, AL, pp. 300–307, 1981.
22. Morrison, A. W.: Endolymphatic Mastoid Shunt for Ménière's Disease. In: Neurological Surgery of the Ear and Skull Base, D. E. Brackmann, (Ed). Raven, New York, pp. 291–297, 1982.
23. Pennington, C. L. and Stevens, E. L.: Ultrasonic Ablation of the Labyrinth in the Treatment of Endolymphatic Hypertension (Ménière's Disease). S. Med. J., 60:34–43, 1967.
24. Pennington, C. L., Stevens, E. L., and Griffin, W. L.: The Use of Ultrasound in the Treatment of Ménière's Disease. Laryngoscope, 80:578–598, 1970.
25. Portmann, G.: Vertigo Surgical Treatment by Opening the Saccus Endolymphaticus. Arch. Otolaryngol., 6:309–315, 1927.
26. Pulec, J. L.: The Otic-Perotic Shunt. Otolaryngol. Clin. N. Am., 1:643–648, 1968.
27. Schuknecht, H. F.: Ablation Therapy for the Relief of Ménière's Disease. Laryngoscope, 66:859–870, 1956.
28. Schuknecht, H. F.: Behavior of the Vestibular Nerve Following Labyrinthectomy. Ann. Otol. Rhinol. Laryngol., 91(suppl. 97):16–32.

29. Schucknecht, H. F.: Cochleosacculotomy for Méniére's Disease: Theory, Technique, and Results. *Laryngoscope*, 92:853–858, 1982.

30. Shambaugh, G. E., Jr., Clemis, J. D., and Arenberg, I. K.: Endolymphatic Duct and Sac in Méniére's Disease. *Arch. Otolaryngol.*, 89:816–825, 1969.

31. Shea, J. J.: Teflon Film Drainage of the Endolymphatic Sac. *Arch. Otolaryngol.*, 83:316–319, 1966.

32. Silverstein, H.: Partial or Total Eighth Nerve Section in the Treatment of Vertigo. In: Neurological Surgery of the Ear, Vol. II, H. Silverstein and H. Norrell (Eds). Aesculapius, Birmingham, AL, pp. 93–103, 1979.

33. Silverstein, H. and Norrell, H.: Retrolabyrinthine Surgery: A Direct Approach to the Cerebellopontine Angle. In: Neurologic Surgery of the Ear, Vol. II, H. Silverstein, and H. Norrell (Eds). Aesculapius, Birmingham, AL, pp. 318–322, 1977.

34. Tabb, H. G., Norris, C. H., and Hogan, W. G.: Round Window Ultrasonic Irradiation for Méniére's Disease with ENG Monitoring. *Laryngoscope*, 88:1460–1467, 1978.

35. Wolfson, R. J., Cutt, R. A., and Ishiyama, E.: Cryosurgery of the Labyrinth—Preliminary Report of a New Surgical Procedure. *Laryngoscope*, 76:733–757, 1966.

16

Facial Nerve Disorders

BELL'S PALSY

WITHOUT LABYRINTHINE INVOLVEMENT

Transmastoid Decompression

A simple mastoidectomy is first performed. The horizontal canal and fossa incudis are identified. Care is exercised not to injure the short process of the incus. The facial nerve is first identified just inferior to the horizontal canal. The mastoid segment of the facial nerve is skeletonized, using first a cutting and then a large diamond burr (Figure 16-1). Exposure extends to the stylomastoid foramen. Bone is removed from slightly more than the lateral half of the nerve. In uncovering the facial nerve, gentle drilling parallel to the course of the nerve is preferred.

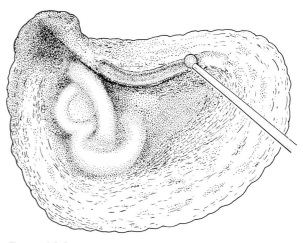

Figure 16-1

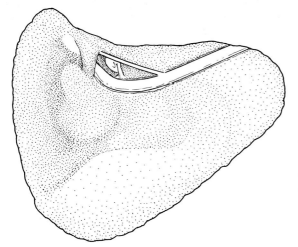

Figure 16-2

Bone is then removed to expose the facial recess (chorda facial angle), allowing visualization of the entire tympanic segment of the nerve to the cochleariformis process, as well as the chorda tympani nerve and stapes (Figure 16-2). Removal of the thin bone covering the tympanic segment of the nerve can best be performed with a slightly blunt pick.

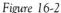

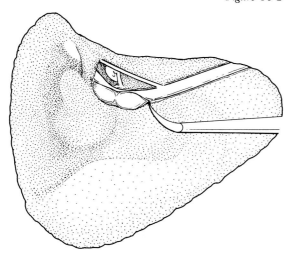

Figure 16-3

By use of small sharp blades, the outermost sheath of the nerve is incised from the cochleariformis process to the stylomastoid foramen (Figure 16-3). By thinning the bar of bone forming the superior base of the chorda facial angle and by rotating the operating table away from the surgeon, it is usually possible to gain greater exposure than is demonstrated in Figure 16-3, thereby allowing complete incision of the sheath to the cochleariformis process. If this is not possible, the incudostapedial joint may be incised and the incus temporarily dislocated for exposure or removed completely from the operative field. At the end of the procedure the incus is replaced in its normal position, supported by Gelfoam.

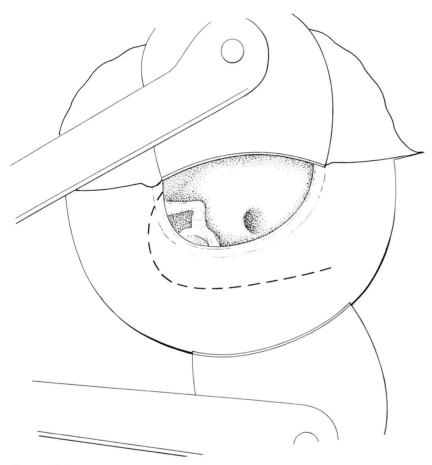

Figure 16-4

Transcanal Facial Nerve Decompression (Meurman,[2] Pou[3])

An alternative approach is through a transcanal exposure using an endaural incision and anterior displacement of the tympanomeatal flap. Bone is removed from the area outlined in Figure 16-4, including exposure of the full extent of the mastoid segment of the facial nerve.

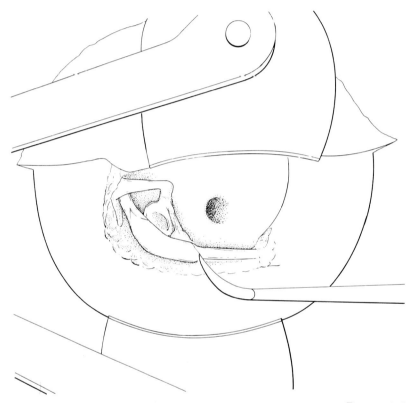

Figure 16-5

In Figure 16-5 the nerve sheath is incised as described earlier. (*Note:* Although simple decompression of the nerve without incision of the sheath has been advocated, the author recommends that the sheath be incised.)

WITH LABYRINTHINE
INVOLVEMENT

Combined Transmastoid–Middle
Fossa Decompression
(House,[1] Pulec[4])

First a postauricular incision is made, a simple mastoidectomy performed, and the mastoid segment of the facial nerve skeletonized as shown in Figure 16-1. It is not necessary to expose the tympanic segment at this time. It is helpful, however, to remove a small circle of bone from the tegmen of the mastoid to use for identification during middle fossa exposure. The postauricular incision is now extended superiorly and anteriorly above the auricle and extended into the middle fossa skin incision previously described in Figure 15-38. Middle fossa exposure is accomplished as described and illustrated in Figures 15-38, 15-39. The facial nerve may be identified either by picking up the greater superficial petrosal nerve at the facial hiatus (see arrow in Figure 16-6) and following it with a diamond burr to the geniculate ganglion, or by visualizing the tympanic segment through the bony defect in the mastoid tegmen created previously. The facial nerve is decompressed distally in its tympanic segment and proximally in its labyrinthine and internal auditory canal segments.

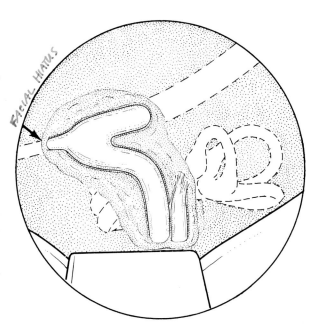

Figure 16-6

The sheath of the nerve is incised from the porus acousticus to the mastoid genu, producing continuity with the incision of the sheath performed through the mastoid (Figure 16-7).

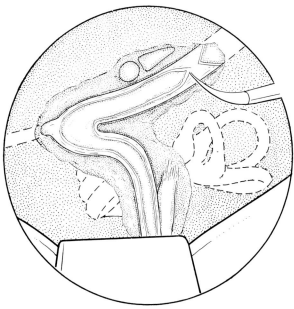

Figure 16-7

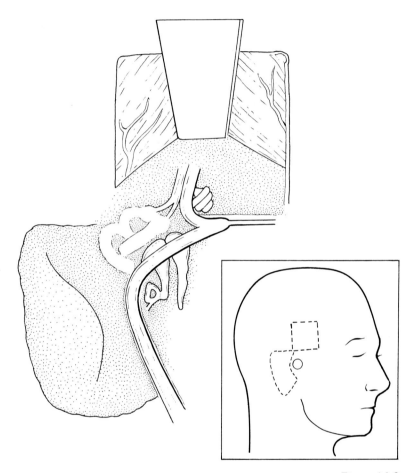

Figure 16-8

The composite illustration shown in Figure 16-8 demonstrates the combined approach to the facial nerve, allowing complete exposure of the nerve from the porus acousticus to the stylomastoid foramen.

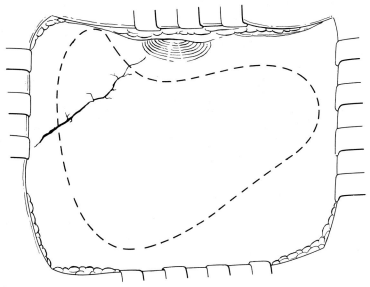

Figure 16-9

TRAUMA

WITHOUT LABYRINTHINE INVOLVEMENT OR SENSORINEURAL LOSS

Transmastoid Decompression

The mastoid space is outlined as shown in Figure 16-9, and a fracture line is also shown, demonstrating the usual alignment of the fracture, centered on the posterosuperior quadrant of the bony ear canal.

A simple mastoidectomy is performed as shown in Figure 16-10, following the fracture into the temporal bone.

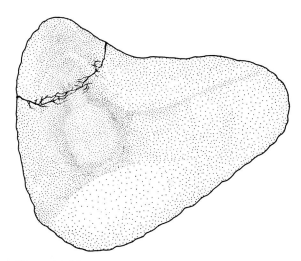

Figure 16-10

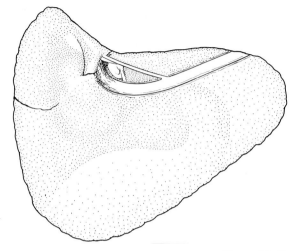

Figure 16-11

Figure 16-11 demonstrates that the fracture line does not involve the bony labyrinth, but has resulted in trauma to the facial nerve at the mastoid genu. The facial recess has been developed as described in Figure 16-2. The nerve is decompressed and the sheath incised as illustrated and described in Figure 16-3. Damage to the ossicular chain is frequently associated with this type of injury and may be repaired using appropriate methods. (*Note:* If the nerve has been transected, repair should consist of sharp resection of devitalized tissue and placement of a nerve graft, using the greater auricular nerve. The graft may be placed in approximation to the severed ends of the facial nerve within the fallopian canal without sutures.)

WITH LABYRINTHINE INVOLVEMENT, NO SENSORINEURAL HEARING LOSS

This situation implies that the fracture line is longitudinal in type, with damage to the facial nerve but without damage to the labyrinth itself, or to the eighth cranial nerve.

Combined Transmastoid–Middle Fossa Decompression (House,[1] Pulec[4])

In Figure 16-12 note the fracture line producing direct injury to the facial nerve, with extensive swelling. Surgical treatment is as described and illustrated in Figures 16-6–16-8. If the nerve is transected, refer to Figure 16-15.

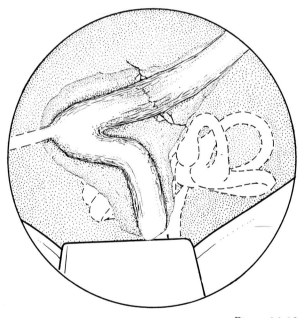

Figure 16-12

WITH LABYRINTHINE INVOLVEMENT AND SENSORINEURAL HEARING LOSS

This situation implies that the fracture is transverse in type, with damage to the facial nerve, as well as to the labyrinth and/or the eighth nerve.

Translabyrinthine Decompression of the Facial Nerve

Because hearing is not a factor, the more simplified translabyrinthine approach is preferred to a middle fossa approach. This is particularly appropriate because balance is very likely to be impaired and thus a labyrinthectomy is indicated. In Figure 16-13 note that a labyrinthectomy has been performed, and the internal auditory canal has been exposed, the dura incised, and the superior and inferior vestibular nerves exposed.

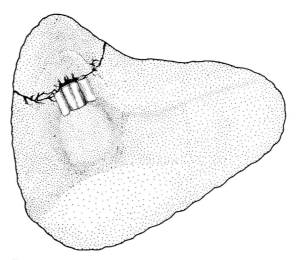

Figure 16-13

The superior and inferior vestibular nerves have been elevated, exposing the facial nerve. As shown in Figure 16-14, the labyrinthine segment of the facial nerve has been completely skeletonized by means of a diamond burr, demonstrating swelling of the nerve. If the nerve is intact, the sheath may simply be incised.

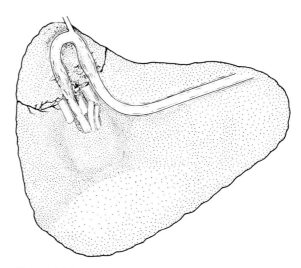

Figure 16-14

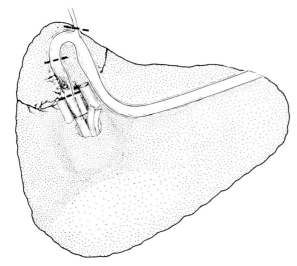

The damage shown in Figure 16-15 is more severe, and the nerve tissue is devitalized. In such a situation, it may be advisable to transect the devitalized segment, as well as the greater superficial petrosal branch (to gain added length).

Figure 16-15

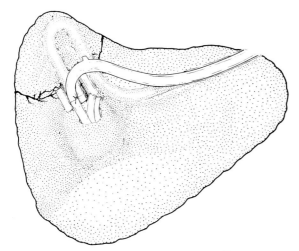

The ends of the nerve may now be approximated using two or three single sutures of 8-0 or 10-0 monofilament nylon (Figure 16-16). If too great a gap is involved, a graft taken from the greater auricular nerve may be interposed.

Figure 16-16

DISCUSSION

Fisch prefers to begin the operation illustrated in Figures 16-6–16-8 by using the middle fossa approach because of his belief that the primary site of pathology is frequently the labyrinthine segment. Many surgeons express skepticism, either stated or implied, over the necessity for decompression of the nerve central to the tympanic segment. They thus limit exposure of the nerve to the mastoid and tympanic segments alone unless obvious edema of the nerve extends centrally and beyond the most anterior exposure of the tympanic segment. Although this is a controversial subject and absolute data are not available, when there are preoperative diagnostic data indicating labyrinthine involvement, the preponderance of experienced opinion is that the entire nerve should be decompressed.

REFERENCES

1. House, W. F.: Surgical Exposure of the Internal Auditory Canal and Its Contents Through the Middle Cranial Fossa. *Laryngoscope,* 71:1363–1385, 1961.
2. Meurman, O. H.: Endaural Tympanic Approach to the Facial Nerve. *Acta Oto-Laryngologica,* 49:495, 1958.
3. Pou, J. W.: Decompression of the Facial Nerve—A Simplified Technique. *Trans. Am. Acad. Ophthalmol. Otolaryngol.,* 72:789–795, 1968.
4. Pulec, J.: Total Decompression of the Facial Nerve. *Laryngoscope,* 76:1015–1028, 1966.

17

Temporal Bone Tumors

GLOMUS TUMORS

TYMPANIC TYPE

This designation includes those glomus tumors arising from glomus bodies located within the tympanic cavity and usually involving Jacobson's nerve.

Confined to the Middle Ear

Transcanal removal. Those tumors clearly confined to the middle ear, and without extension into the mastoid space, may be removed through a transcanal approach. Figure 17-1 shows that a tympanomeatal flap has been elevated and an incision made through the periosteum of the handle of the malleus to allow exposure as required anteriorly.

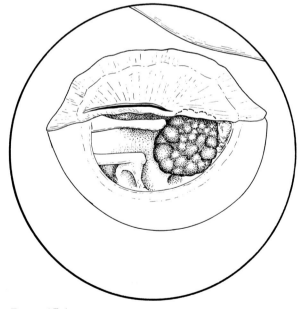

Figure 17-1

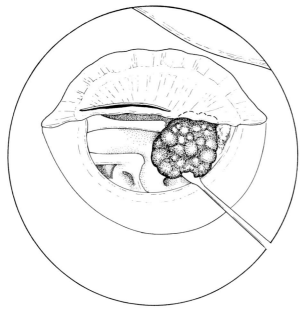

The margins of the tumor are very carefully and bluntly mobilized (Figure 17-2), sufficient only to allow cotton pledgets moistened in an epinephrine-containing solution to be packed around the base of the tumor as a tamponade. Care must be taken to avoid injury to the stapes and facial nerve.

Figure 17-2

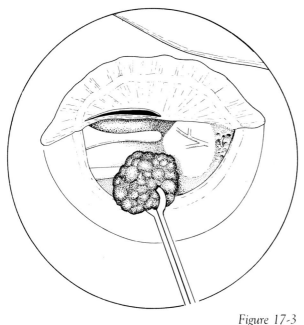

The base of the tumor, which is relatively narrow, is identified, incised, and the tumor removed (Figure 17-3). The base of the tumor frequently extends into the bony surface of the promontory or hypotympanum and should be curetted. Bleeding should have resolved following this. The area may be packed with Gelfoam and the tympanomeatal flap replaced.

Figure 17-3

Extension into the Mastoid Space

Transmastoid removal. Tumor extension into the mastoid space is shown in Figure 17-4. Note extension both through the facial recess (lateral to the facial nerve, which is shown skeletonized) and through the retrofacial air cells (medial to the facial nerve). In this situation the transcanal approach should be combined with simple mastoidectomy. The author prefers first to expose the middle-ear portion of the tumor through a postauricular, transcanal approach, and to mobilize and tamponade the tumor as illustrated earlier in Figures 17-1 and 17-2. Simple mastoidectomy is then carried out.

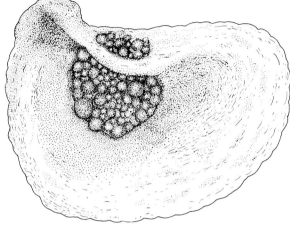

Figure 17-4

If the tumor is extensive, it is usually necessary to drill carefully with a diamond burr and extend the facial recess inferiorly (with sacrifice of the chorda tympani nerve) as well as the retrofacial space (both shown in Figure 17-5). This bone removal allows establishment of a clear inferior margin of the tumor and is illustrated in Figure 17-5.

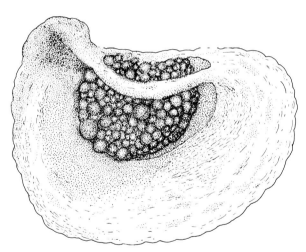

Figure 17-5

JUGULARE TYPE

Glomus jugulare tumors originate from glomus bodies located on the dome of the jugular bulb, in the jugular fossa. They almost invariably produce blockage of the bulb and frequently involve the lower cranial nerves and extend into the middle ear and mastoid. They also may involve the facial nerve and occasionally involve the internal carotid artery and the posterior cranial fossa.

Combined Approach to the Skull Base[2–4]

Figure 17-6 shows that a right postauricular skin incision has been made and extended into the upper neck. The membranous ear canal has been transected. The facial nerve is first identified at the stylomastoid foramen and followed peripherally into the parotid gland, which is shown on the right. Soft-tissue structures are resected from the base of the skull to the posterior lip of the jugular foramen. The sternocleidomastoid muscle is shown reflected inferiorly. The internal jugular vein and internal carotid artery are shown entering the skull base, along with cranial nerves 9–12. A simple mastoidectomy is performed, skeletonizing the mastoid segment of the facial nerve, as shown, and demonstrating any extension of the tumor into the mastoid. In Figure 17-6 tumor tissue is seen in the facial recess. The upper portion of the sigmoid sinus has been skeletonized, using a large diamond burr.

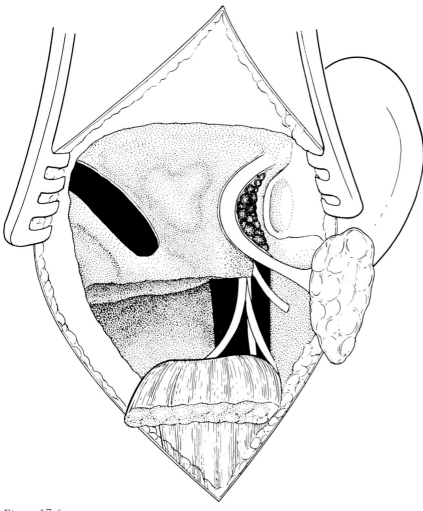

Figure 17-6

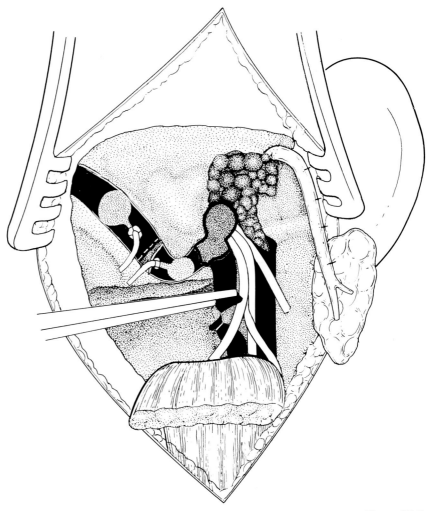

Figure 17-7

In Figure 17-7 bone removal has been continued with resection of the bony ear canal and the bone overlying the inferior portion of the sigmoid sinus and jugular bulb, including the bone of the posterior half of the jugular foramen. To allow this, the facial nerve has been elevated from the fallopian canal and transposed anteriorly into a soft-tissue bed. The jugular bulb, containing the primary tumor mass, is seen in the center of Figure 17-7 with tumor extending superiorly into the area of the tympanum. The internal jugular vein has been ligated and divided. The sigmoid sinus has been occluded proximally and distally with Fogarty venous catheters as shown, allowing division of the lateral wall of the sinus with closure by imbrication distally as shown.

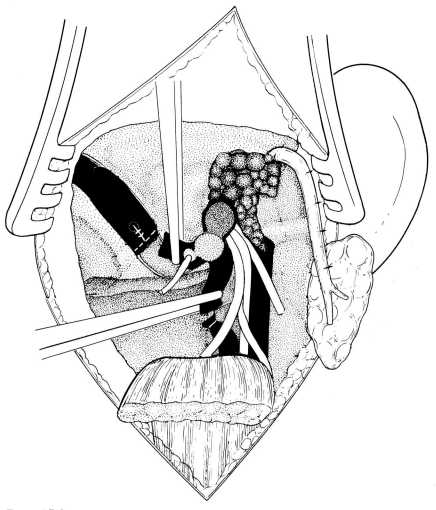

Figure 17-8

In Figure 17-8 the catheter in the distal segment of the sigmoid sinus has been removed and its pursestring suture closed. The tumor specimen is ready for en bloc removal. The internal carotid artery is seen and is not significantly involved.

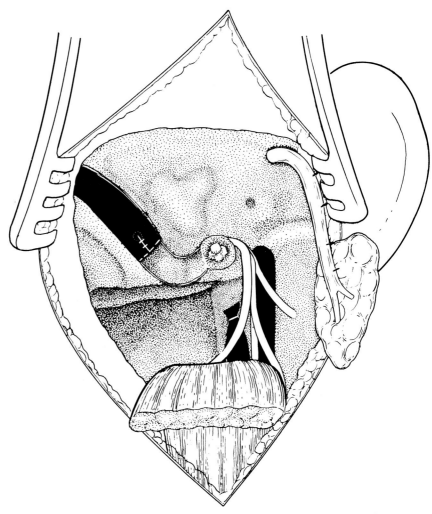

Figure 17-9

In Figure 17-9 the tumor has been removed. Packing is seen in the lumen of the inferior petrosal sinus. The membranous ear canal is removed with the tumor. We agree with Fisch that the mastoid space should be obliterated and the ear canal closed at the meatus. The facial nerve is left in its anteriorly displaced position. A groove drilled vertically along the anterior attic wall, as described by Fisch, facilitates this. Abdominal adipose tissue is used to fill the operative site and the wound closed primarily in layers.

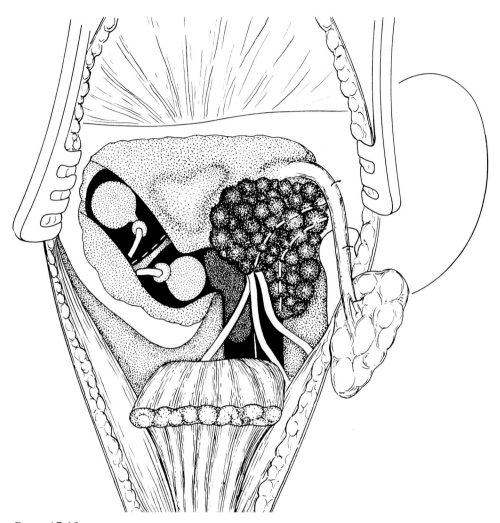

Figure 17-10

Figure 17-10 illustrates a glomus jugulare tumor extending anteriorly and involving the internal carotid artery, which is shown by dotted lines surrounded by tumor. In this situation we either resect the mandibular ramus or retract it anteriorly, allowing the bone of the anterior ear canal and tympanum, the bone of the temporomandibular joint to be drilled away, and the anterior tumor extension and carotid artery thereby exposed. In such circumstances we have not found it necessary to resect the carotid but have encountered a tear in the vessel on one occasion that we were able to repair with arterial suture. Extension of such a tumor into the posterior fossa has been managed through the skull base exposure described previously, removing this portion of the tumor with the primary tumor mass. In such situations we have found the intracranial portion of the tumor to be extradural, and the dura has been found to be intact, even in the presence of very large extension into the posterior fossa.

CEREBELLOPONTINE ANGLE TUMORS

The great majority of these tumors are acoustic tumors and present with otologic complaints. Surgical treatment varies depending on tumor size. Generally speaking, very small tumors in patients having good hearing in the involved ear may be removed through a middle fossa approach; larger tumors, and small tumors in patients having poor hearing in the involved ear, are removed through a translabyrinthine approach; and very large tumors are removed through a combined translabyrinthine and suboccipital approach. The limiting factor for use of the middle fossa approach is that the cerebellopontine portion of the tumor must be no greater than approximately 1 cm; and for use of the translabyrinthine approach, that the neurosurgeon feel comfortable, based on personal experience, with tumor removal through this approach.

TRANSLABYRINTHINE APPROACH

In the case shown in Figure 17-11 a simple mastoidectomy has been completed. The middle and posterior fossa dural plates, sigmoid sinus, and jugular bulb are skeletonized. The incus has been removed, the malleus head is seen, and a labyrinthectomy has been performed as illustrated in Figures 15-7–15-9. The internal auditory canal is skeletonized by removal of bone from the superior, posterior, and inferior lips of the canal. The posterior fossa dura anterior to the sigmoid sinus is skeletonized as shown. The cribriform areas of the horizontal and superior semicircular canals are used as guides to the superior vestibular nerve canal, which is skeletonized at the lateral end of the internal auditory canal. The dural covering of the canal has been incised and opened, exposing the superior vestibular nerve.

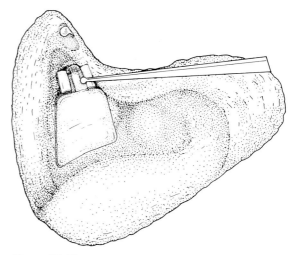

Figure 17-11

In Figure 17-12 the most lateral fibers of the superior vestibular nerve are elevated, revealing the vertical crest of the internal auditory canal (see upper arrow), beneath which lies the facial nerve (see lower arrow).

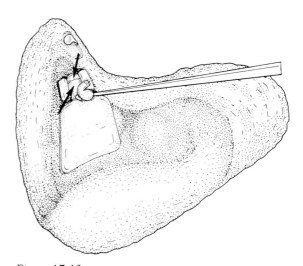

Figure 17-12

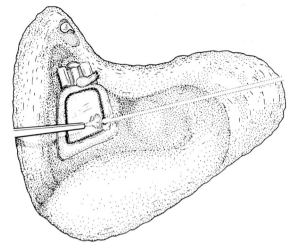

A carbon dioxide (CO_2) laser beam is shown on the right in Figure 17-13 vaporizing the dura overlying the posterior fossa. A suction tip is shown on the left removing the resulting plume of smoke.

Figure 17-13

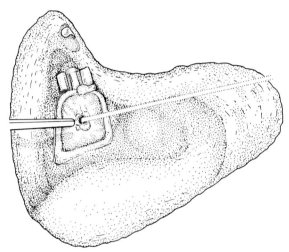

In Figure 17-14 the dura has been elevated and removed, and the tumor is now seen in the cerebellopontine angle. The CO_2 laser is again being used, now to vaporize the tumor itself as debulking of the tumor is begun.

Figure 17-14

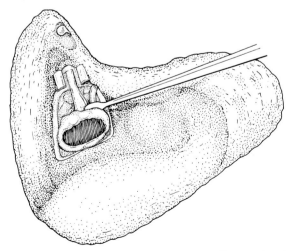

After the tumor has been reduced in size to approximately 1 cm, or when the root entry zones of cranial nerves 7 and 8 are approached during posterior dissection of the tumor, development of the anterior tumor plane is begun, elevating the tumor from the surface of the facial nerve on the left and from the cochlear division of the eighth nerve on the right (Figure 17-15).

Figure 17-15

In Figure 17-16 the tumor has been removed. The facial nerve is seen on the left to be intact but typically thinned. The cochlear division, seldom directly involved by the tumor, is seen on the right. The cochlear division is resected.

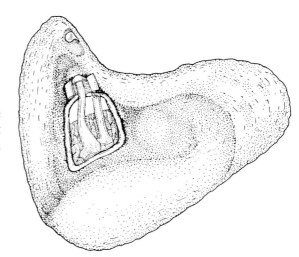

Figure 17-16

Rectus abdominus fascia is placed over the opening into the cerebellopontine angle (Figure 17-17). Muscle tissue and Proplast (Dow Corning) are placed in the attic, additus, and vestibule. Abdominal adipose tissue is used to fill the mastoid cavity firmly in order to maintain the fascia tightly in position over the opening in the angle. The wound is closed in layers.

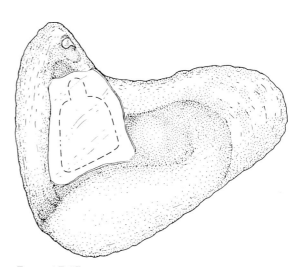

Figure 17-17

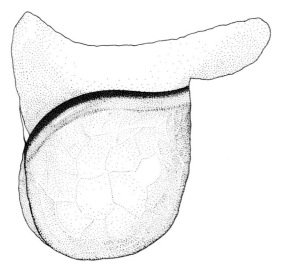

COMBINED TRANSLABYRINTHINE-SUBOCCIPITAL APPROACH

In Figure 17-18 the tumor has been exposed anteriorly through the translabyrinthine approach, shown without details in the upper part of the illustration, and with detail in preceding illustrations (see Figures 17-11–17-15). In Figure 17-18 the sigmoid sinus is seen skeletonized in the center, and the dura overlying the cerebellum is shown in the lower portion.

Figure 17-18

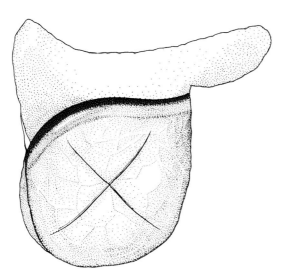

Figure 17-19 shows incision of the dura overlying the cerebellum.

Figure 17-19

In Figure 17-20 the dura has been elevated and retracted (see traction sutures), and the underlying cerebellum exposed.

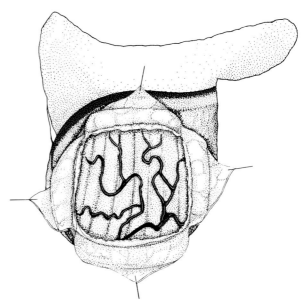

Figure 17-20

In Figure 17-21 the cerebellum is being retracted, revealing the tumor filling the cerebellopontine angle.

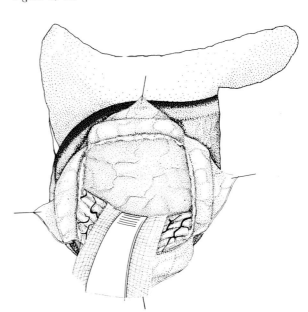

Figure 17-21

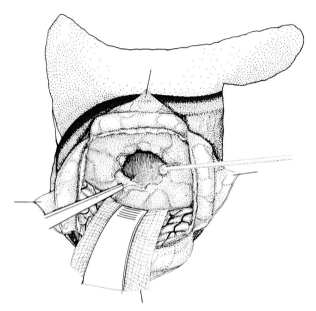

In Figure 17-22 the tumor is being reduced in size by using the CO_2 laser. The tumor extends posterior to and beneath the sigmoid sinus.

Figure 17-22

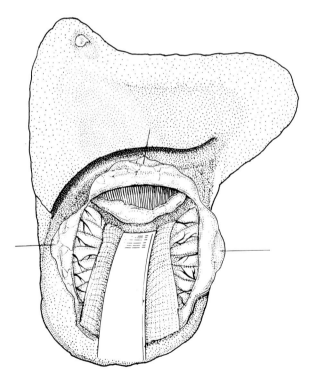

Figure 17-23 shows the tumor capsule being elevated superiorly, posteriorly, and inferiorly, with the tumor substance gradually reducing in size as shown here.

Figure 17-23

In Figure 17-24 the remaining tumor mass has been pushed forward into the mastoid cavity, where it is shown undergoing final removal. The facial nerve and cochlear nerve are shown intact.

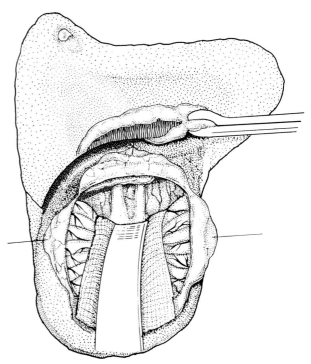

Figure 17-24

In Figure 17-25 the dura is shown closed, with rectus abdominus fascia placed over the translabyrinthine opening into the angle, muscle placed into the attic, and Proplast wedged into the additus as shown.

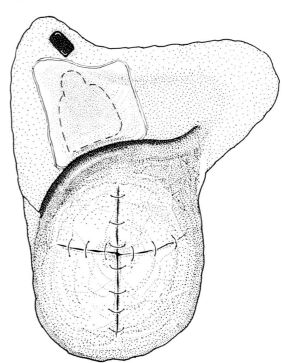

Figure 17-25

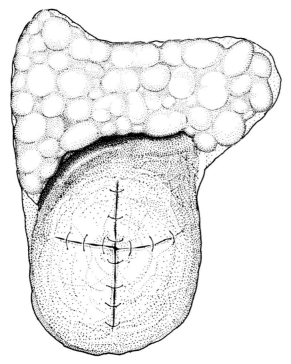

The mastoid space is filled with several large pieces of adipose tissue (Figure 17-26). This is packed fairly tightly to maintain firm approximation of the underlying fascia.

Figure 17-26

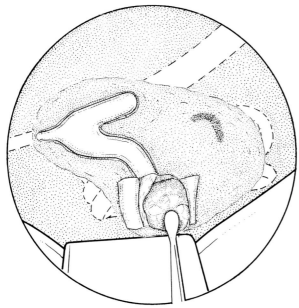

Figure 17-27

MIDDLE FOSSA APPROACH

The middle fossa approach was illustrated previously (see Figures 15-38–15-41 and 16-6). The bone over the internal auditory canal is widely removed, skeletonizing the superior semicircular canal as shown in Figure 17-27. The greater superficial petrosal nerve is identified and followed by drilling carefully over it with a diamond burr to the geniculate ganglion, and the facial nerve is then followed into the middle ear and internal auditory canal as shown. Care is taken not to open the cochlea or superior semicircular canal. When adequate bony exposure has been accomplished, the dura of the internal canal is incised, and the tumor is visualized as shown. Note the facial nerve displaced anteriorly. The tumor is removed by using a combination of the CO_2 laser and conventional dissection. Great care must be taken to avoid injury to the vasculature of the internal canal. Before closing the wound, all exposed air cells are sealed with bone wax. Temporalis muscle and fascia are placed over the bony defect and the wound closed in layers.

ALTERNATIVE APPROACHES

Suboccipital Approach

After the tumor has been reduced in size sufficiently, or initially with a smaller tumor as shown in Figure 17-28, dura is resected from over the bone of the petrous pyramid covering the internal auditory canal. The patient is in the recumbent position, and the tumor is on the right side. A rotating burr is being used to expose the tumor occupying the internal auditory canal. Cranial nerves 9–12 are seen to the right, inferiorly.

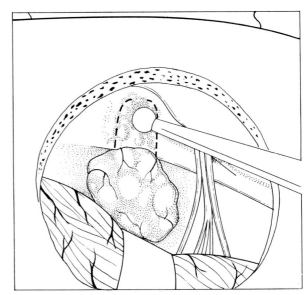

Figure 17-28

Following skeletonization of the canal, the dura is incised from the porus acousticus medially to the lateral end of the canal, exposing the tumor (Figure 17-29).

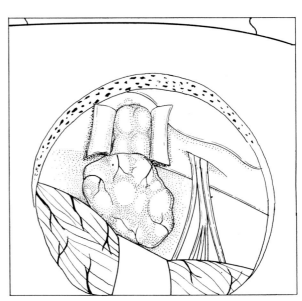

Figure 17-29

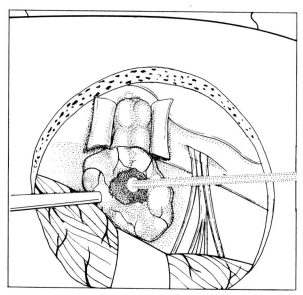

Figure 17-30

The CO_2 laser is used to vaporize the tumor and thereby reduce its size (Figure 17-30). Tumor removal is carried out, developing a plane between the tumor and the facial nerve, which lies "beneath" the tumor, or anteriorly to it. Muscle is placed into the bony defect, fascia is placed over this, and the wound is closed in layers.

Retrocochlear Approach

This approach to the cerebellopontine angle, from anterior to the sigmoid sinus with preservation of the labyrinth, was illustrated in Figures 15-42 and 15-43. It has been used as an alternative to the translabyrinthine approach when bilateral tumors are present, in an effort to save hearing in one or both ears.

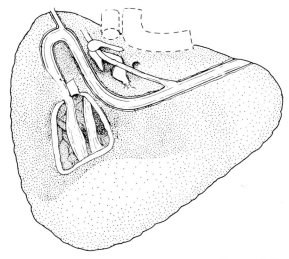

Figure 17-31

Transcochlear Approach
(House and Hitselberger[5])

This approach has great merit for exposure of a tumor extending well anteriorly in the cerebellopontine angle, such as a large meningioma or a chordoma. In Figure 17-31 a labyrinthectomy has been performed, the entire facial nerve decompressed, and the internal auditory canal opened. The middle-ear structures are seen, and the eustachian tube and internal carotid artery are shown with dotted lines. The tumor is seen "beneath," or anterior to the facial nerve.

In Figure 17-32 the chorda tympani and greater superficial petrosal nerves have been incised and the facial nerve elevated from the fallopian canal and transposed posteriorly.

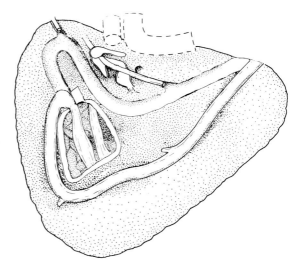

Figure 17-32

In Figure 17-33 a rotating burr has been used to drill away the bone of the vestibule, cochlea, and bony eustachian tube, thereby widely exposing the tumor and adjacent internal carotid artery and allowing tumor removal. The dura on which the tumor is based may be cauterized prior to removal through this procedure, allowing less bleeding.

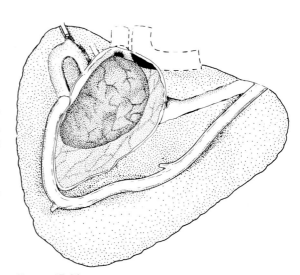

Figure 17-33

MALIGNANT TUMORS

TEMPORAL BONE RESECTION

This procedure implies the presence of a proven malignant tumor of the temporal bone with involvement beyond the ear canal and tympanic membrane into the middle ear, with presumed involvement of the bone of the labyrinth. Nothing less than radical resection of the temporal bone is likely to benefit the patient. The area of resection includes the skin and mucous membrane-lined portions of the temporal bone, with adjacent margins extending to the posterior fossa dura posteriorly, the medial end of the internal auditory canal medially, the internal carotid artery anteriorly, and the dome of the jugular bulb inferiorly. A variety of surgical approaches must be employed.

The right temporal bone is viewed laterally in Figure 17-34. The tumor is seen centrally within the temporal bone (see arrow), extending out the ear canal. The middle fossa structures are seen ghosted in. Skin incisions have been made. That portion of the auricle not involved by tumor is judiciously preserved. Soft-tissue structures have been resected from the base of the skull to the lip of the jugular foramen. The carotid artery and lower cranial nerves are visualized. The facial nerve is identified at the stylomastoid foramen, followed into the parotid gland and divided as shown. The zygomatic arch is divided. The ramus of the mandible is resected and the temporomandibular joint space exposed. With the use of an electrically driven burr, posterior fossa dura and sigmoid sinus are skeletonized posteriorly. The exposure extends to the lip of the jugular foramen, and the internal carotid artery is skeletonized from the lip of the carotid foramen in the base of the skull to its major genu. The eustachian tube is resected at the latter level as shown, and the lumen is examined carefully for tumor involvement. (Note: Soft-tissue exposure at the base of the skull is critical to the success of this procedure and requires a creative effort on the part of the surgeon.)

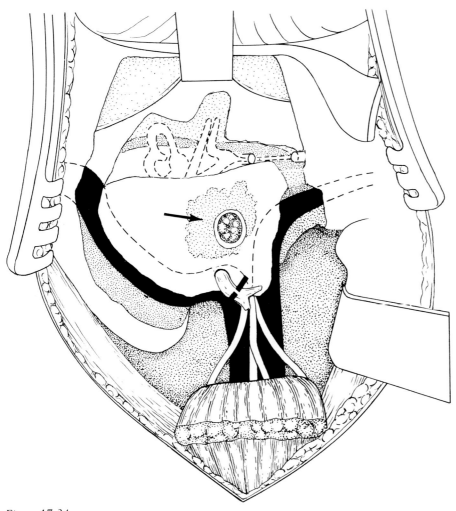

Figure 17-34

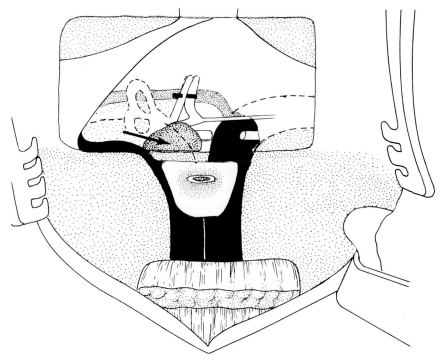

Figure 17-35

In Figure 17-35 the patient's head is repositioned to allow middle fossa exploration. The extension that is desirable during soft-tissue exposure of the skull base is now converted to lateral flexion of the head on the neck. Middle fossa exposure is carried out as illustrated in Figures 15-39–41 and 16-6. In this illustration (Figure 17-35) the tumor is seen within the depths of the temporal bone (see arrow) and overlies the jugular bulb. The eustachian tube is shown divided. With the use of a rotating burr, the internal auditory canal is opened at its lateral end. The seventh and eighth cranial nerves are cauterized and sectioned, and bone wax is placed in the medial lumen of the canal. Care is taken to avoid injury to any vascular loop present within the canal. The cut across the canal (see dark dotted lines) is now extended posteriorly to the dura of the posterior fossa and anteriorly to the internal carotid artery. The same bone cut is extended deeply (inferiorly) to the dome of the jugular bulb, thereby completing the cut across the petrous apex. If this cut is not made completely through the bone, from soft tissue to soft tissue, mobilization of the tumor specimen will very likely produce damage to the cranial nerves in the jugular foramen.

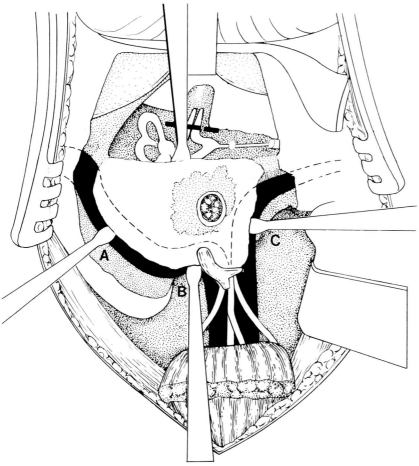

Figure 17-36

Figure 17-36 shows the following maneuvers, with the use of elevators: (A) posteriorly, the dura of the posterior fossa is carefully stripped away from the posterior surface of the specimen; (B) inferiorly, the lower sigmoid sinus and jugular bulb are elevated away; and (C) anteriorly, the carotid artery is also elevated from the specimen. The tumor specimen should be free for removal. Temporalis muscle is rotated into the cavity, and abdominal adipose tissue is used to complete cavity obliteration. The wound is closed in layers. Any tears in the dura are repaired.

SUBTOTAL TEMPORAL BONE RESECTION

When a malignant tumor involves only the ear canal, a less radical procedure may be employed. The skull base is exposed as shown in Figure 17-34. The facial nerve is identified at the stylomastoid foramen and preserved. The zygomatic arch is divided as shown in Figure 17-34. The ramus of the mandible is resected or retracted anteriorly, and the temporomandibular joint space is exposed. A simple mastoidectomy is performed, along with demonstration of the extended facial recess. The internal carotid artery is skeletonized anteriorly. The extended facial recess cut is further extended anteriorly to make contact with the carotid artery exposure. The tumor specimen is now able to be removed. Routine mastoid closure is carried out.

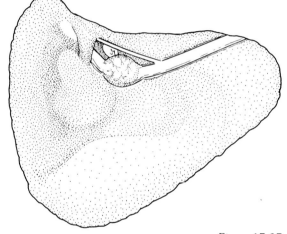

Figure 17-37

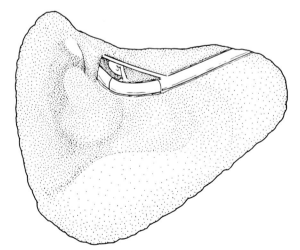

Figure 17-38

FACIAL NERVE NEUROMA

A neuroma of the facial nerve is shown in Figure 17-37 involving the genu. In fact, such a tumor can occur at any point along the course of the facial nerve, requiring a variety of surgical approaches. In this instance a simple mastoidectomy is performed and bone removed from around the tumor, opening the facial recess. The tumor is then resected with adequate margins.

Figure 17-38 shows a nerve graft taken from the greater auricular nerve being interposed in the defect. Sutures are not required.

DISCUSSION

Occasionally a tympanic tumor may be quite extensive, with erosion into the labyrinth, involvement of the facial nerve, deep penetration into the hypotympanum, and involvement of the internal carotid artery. In these situations, careful preoperative evaluation with computerized tomography (CT) scan and arteriography to rule out a glomus jugulare tumor and individualization of surgical approach are necessary. Shambaugh and Farrior have described a hypotympanotomy approach that is useful. It is important to have adequate exposure for complete tumor removal. In removing bone from around the tumor, it is important to use a large diamond burr. When bleeding occurs in one area, Gelfoam may be left in place and attention directed elsewhere until bleeding has slowed. The temptation to begin tumor removal piecemeal prior to adequate exposure of the complete tumor should be avoided.

Several principles underlie the combined approach to the skull base for removal of glomus jugulare tumors (Figures 17-6–17-10). We believe that irradiation therapy has a significant effect on many of these tumors and may be employed for reduction of vascularity prior to surgical removal, or as a primary form of therapy. Surgery is made difficult by the tumor's relative inaccessibility to conventional surgical approach, its vascular nature, and its proximity to important neurovascular structures. Surgery by incremental removal of the tumor leads to incomplete removal and the risk of recurrence. Surgical resection is feasible but requires wide skull base exposure through a cooperative team effort and is benefited by preoperative irradiation therapy and occasionally by preoperative embolization. En bloc removal of the entire tumor mass including its attached venous structures is desirable. Younger individuals, and older individuals in good medical condition in whom tumor growth is not controlled by irradiation, are considered to be surgical candidates. Older patients who are not suitable medical risks or who demonstrate control of tumor growth by irradiation therapy are not treated surgically, based on our experience. Older patients whose tumors are not controlled by irradiation but who are not surgical candidates because of poor general health

may be candidates for embolization without surgery.

Many alternative approaches have been described in the literature on the subject illustrated in Figure 17-10. The hypotympanotomy approach, as well as the transmastoid approach using the extended facial recess, and illustrated earlier (See Figure 17-5), have been advocated in the past. A purely neurosurgical approach, based on suboccipital exposure has been described frequently in the neurosurgical literature. Skull base exposure without removal of the posterior-ear canal wall has also been advocated, with or without transposition of the facial nerve. We believe that all these alternatives have in common limited access to the tumor, which we feel is undesirable. Fisch[1] has described an infratemporal fossa approach for anterior tumor extension. We assume that the method we discussed with Figure 17-10 is a limited form of this approach and have not required the wider exposure described by Fisch. We believe it ironic that neurosurgeons for many years have been able to resect glomus tumors successfully from the posterior fossa but have felt that extension into the temporal bone was inoperable, whereas during the same timeframe otolaryngologists have had available the methods to deal successfully with glomus tumors of the temporal bone, but have felt that extension into the posterior fossa was inoperable. Combined approach surgery using a team approach now allows composite removal of the entire tumor mass as an en bloc procedure.

The suboccipital approach illustrated in Figures 17-28–17-30 is the traditional neurosurgical technique originally developed by Cushing, Dandy, and others. Its major advantages over the translabyrinthine approach are better exposure of large tumor masses in the cerebellopontine angle and less incidence of cerebrospinal fluid (CSF) leakage postoperatively. Its disadvantages are less direct early visualization of the facial nerve in the lateral end of the internal auditory canal and the necessity of cerebellar retraction. The initial steps of the procedure are seen in Figures 17-18–17-22.

Great care must be taken in use of the high-speed drill over the open operative field. Although some situations favor identification of the facial nerve in the lateral end of the internal auditory canal with this approach, it is not as reliable as the translabyrinthine approach and hence is not used by the author. Very careful technique must be used to avoid cerebellar trauma during retraction. There is great interest at this time in utilizing this approach in an effort to preserve hearing. The author believes that the middle fossa approach is superior in this regard.

Regarding the procedures illustrated in Figures 17-11–17-33, in general, working in the cerebellopontine angle exposes the otolaryngologist to a variety of potential problems that are not ordinarily encountered. Collaboration with a neurosurgical associate is strongly recommended. Great care must be taken to avoid injuries to the important vasculature associated with this area, particularly the anteroinferior cerebellar artery and its branches. Equal care must be applied to the adjacent cerebellum and brain stem. If facial nerve function is to be preserved, the surgeon must avoid all forms of injury to it, particularly catching it in the tip of the suction. Special instrumentation is important in this regard. In all these procedures adequate time must be taken and well-established methods employed to close the wound in order to avoid postoperative CSF leakage. At the present time there is no consensus as to the ideal surgical approach to the cerebellopontine angle. Unfortunately, there have been too many instances in which a particular approach is advocated for traditional or "territorial" reasons. The author believes that the ideal approach in a particular circumstance is one that provides adequate exposure for the circumstances involved, including not only the tumor but also the particular anatomy involved, and the experience and skill of the operating surgeons. The combined approach described in reference to Figures 17-18–17-26 is the preferred approach for larger tumors, in the author's opinion.

REFERENCES

1. Fisch, U.: Infratemporal Fossa Approach for Extensive Tumors of the Temporal Bone and Base of the Skull. In: Neurological Surgery of the Ear, H. Silverstein, and H. Norrell (Eds). Aesculapius, Birmingham, AL, pp. 34–53, 1977.
2. Gardner, G., Cocke, E. W., Robertson, J. T., et al.: Combined Approach Surgery for Removal of Glomus Jugulare Tumors. Laryngoscope, 87:665–688, 1977.
3. Gardner, G., Cocke, E. W., Robertson, J. T., et al.: Glomus Jugulare Tumors—Combined Treatment: Part I. Laryngol. Otol., 95:437–454, 1981.
4. Gardner, G., Cocke, E. W., Robertson, J. T., et al.: Glomus Jugulare Tumors—Combined Treatment: Part II. Laryngol. Otol., 95:567–580, 1981.
5. House, W. F. and Hitselberger, W. E.: The Transcochlear Approach to the Skull Base. Arch. Otolaryngol., 102:334–342, 1976.

Index

Absence
   of incus. *See* Incus, absence of
   of malleus
      congenital, 272
      with incus absence
         and suprastructure of stapes absence, surgical
            reconstruction for, 111–112
         surgical reconstruction for, 110
   of oval window, congenital, 281–285
   of stapes, surgical reconstruction for, 104
   of suprastructure of stapes
      congenital, 274, 276
      with malleus and incus absence, surgical
         reconstruction for, 111–112
Allograft, definition of, 117
Antrotomy and canalplasty for aural atresia, 263–268
Argon laser for stapedectomy, 169–171
Artery, stapedial, persistent, complicating
   stapedectomy, 188
Atresia, aural, 263–271. *See also* Aural atresia
Atticotympanotomy
   combined transcanal and postauricular, for middle-
      ear congenital cholesteatoma, 142–151
   endaural, for middle-ear congenital cholesteatoma,
      142
Auditory canal, external, development of, in embryo,
   262

Aural atresia, 263–271
   canal grafting techniques for, 286–291
   canalplasty for, 269
      with antrotomy, 263–268
      homograft, 271
   mastoidectomy and tympanoplasty for, 270
Auricle
   plastic reconstruction of, prosthetic auricle versus,
      294
   prosthetic, versus plastic auricular reconstruction,
      294
Auricular development in embryo, 262
Autograft, definition of, 117

Balance disorders of labyrinthine origin, 299–324
   with hearing
      from benign paroxysmal positional vertigo in, 317
      from incapacitating vertigo of multiple causes,
         318–321
      from Ménière's disease, 309–316. *See also*
         Ménière's disease
      from round window fistula, 321–322
      surgical management of, 309–322
   with hearing loss
      Day procedure for, 304
      surgical management of, 299–308

a
b
3 c
4 d
5 e
6 f
7 g
8 h
9 i
8 0 j